HEALTH FOR THE PACIFIC 9

Healthy Relationships

in Papua New Guinea

Richard Jones and Jennifer Miller

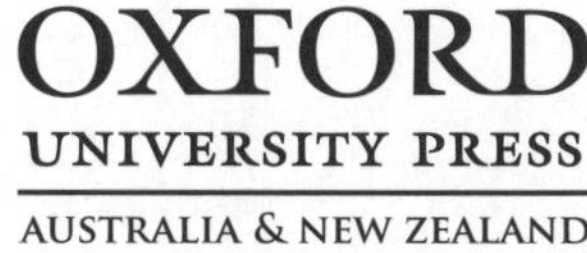

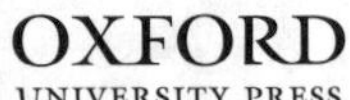

Oxford University Press is a department of the University of Oxford.
It furthers the University's objective of excellence in research,
scholarship, and education by publishing worldwide. Oxford is a registered
trademark of Oxford University Press in the UK and in certain other countries.

Published in Australia by
Oxford University Press
253 Normanby Road, South Melbourne, Victoria 3205, Australia

© Richard Jones and Jennifer Miller 2011
The moral rights of the author have been asserted
First published 2011

All rights reserved. No part of this publication may be reproduced, stored in a retrieval system, or transmitted, in any form or by any means, without the prior permission in writing of Oxford University Press, or as expressly permitted by law, by licence, or under terms agreed with the reprographics rights organisation. Enquiries concerning reproduction outside the scope of the above should be sent to the Rights Department, Oxford University Press, at the address above.

You must not circulate this work in any other form and you must impose this same condition on any acquirer.

ISBN 978 0 19 557596 5

Reproduction and communication for educational purposes

The Australian *Copyright Act 1968* (the Act) allows a maximum of one chapter or 10% of the pages of this work, whichever is the greater, to be reproduced and/or communicated by any educational institution for its educational purposes provided that the educational institution (or the body that administers it) has given a remuneration notice to Copyright Agency Limited (CAL) under the Act.

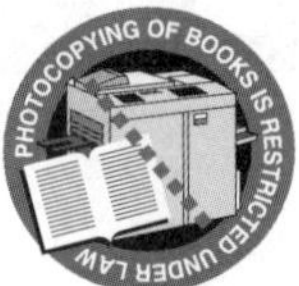

For details of the CAL licence for educational institutions contact:

Copyright Agency Limited
Level 15, 233 Castlereagh Street
Sydney NSW 2000
Telephone: (02) 9394 7600
Facsimile: (02) 9394 7601
Email: info@copyright.com.au

Illustrated by Uramina and Nelson
Typeset by Leigh Ashforth
Proofread by Emma Short
Printed by Golden Cup Printing

Links to third party websites are provided by Oxford in good faith and for information only. Oxford disclaims any responsibility for the materials contained in any third party website referenced in this work.

Contents

Foreword

The *Health for the Pacific* series aims to educate young men and women about important health issues that are affecting their lives.

Throughout a person's life, he or she will have many kinds of relationships with different people. Relationships can bring joy and support, but they can also be a cause of many of the challenges that young people experience. Maintaining healthy relationships with peers, adults and the community is essential. Learning the skills and values that help build successful relationships is an important part of growing up.

This book aims to give accurate and positive information about how to manage, form and change relationships.

Acknowledgments

Teaching about relationships is an important part of educating young people and contributing to their personal development. This text is written to support the teaching of Community Living and Personal Development in primary and secondary schools. It is a textbook for students and a resource book for teachers.

We would like to thank the many dedicated teachers, role models and peer educators who help young people develop and maintain healthy relationships. We also dedicate this book to our friends Jan and Eunice, whose lifelong marriage inspired many of the lessons and advice in this book.

Richard Jones and Jennifer Miller

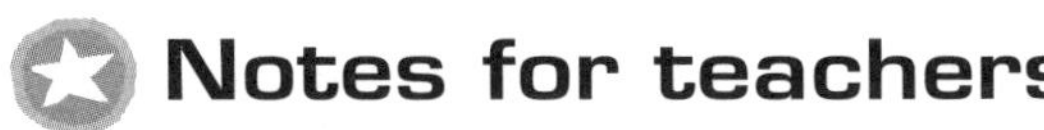

Notes for teachers

This textbook is written to be used by primary and secondary students and their teachers.

The knowledge, skills and attitudes in the text develop these learning outcomes from the Community Living and Personal Development syllabus:

Community Living Grades 3–5

3.1.2 Describe relationships between individuals and groups

4.1.2 Explain behaviour that promotes good relationships in the wider community

5.1.2 Investigate standards of behaviour in different relationships

Personal Development Grades 6–8

6.1.1 Identify groups to which they belong such as family, friends and tribes

7.1.1 Describe different types of families and the roles of family members

8.1.1 Describe standards of behaviour that are important to their community and to families and groups to which they belong

6.1.2 Identify different types of relationships and how people interact with each other

7.1.2 Develop codes of behaviour appropriate to different relationships and groups

8.1.2 Examine the rights of individuals in different forms of relationships

8.1.3 Explain how different ways of describing people influence how people value and treat themselves and others

7.1.5 Demonstrate skills needed to maintain relationships

8.1.5 Describe ways in which relationships form, develop, adapt and end

Personal Development Grades 9–10

9.1.1 Identify factors that determine self concept and self esteem

9.1.2 Explain how their values and attitudes can contribute towards a positive community

9.1.3 Demonstrate skills for establishing and maintaining positive relationships

10.1.3 Compare and contrast the effectiveness of a range of decision-making skills and conflict resolution skills in regard to sexual issues

10.2.1 Explain the importance of peaceful and healthy family values

10.2.2 Identify characteristics of positive peer groups that contribute to class and school spirit

Personal Development Grades 11–12

3 Display positive behaviour as a role model, mentor and advocate showing respect for difference and diversity

4 Demonstrate positive relationship skills and understand the factors that lead to a healthy marriage and good parenting

There are many activities in the text for the students to complete and discuss. These can be used for self study or as teaching and learning activities in class. They are designed for maximum student participation and developing life skills.

Introduction

Relationships are a very important part of people's lives. Young people have relationships with peers, teachers, their family and the community they live in. As young people move from childhood to adulthood, their roles and responsibilities will change. The relationships that young people have with their family, friends and community will also start to change. They will also start to experience new kinds of relationships, including romantic relationships.

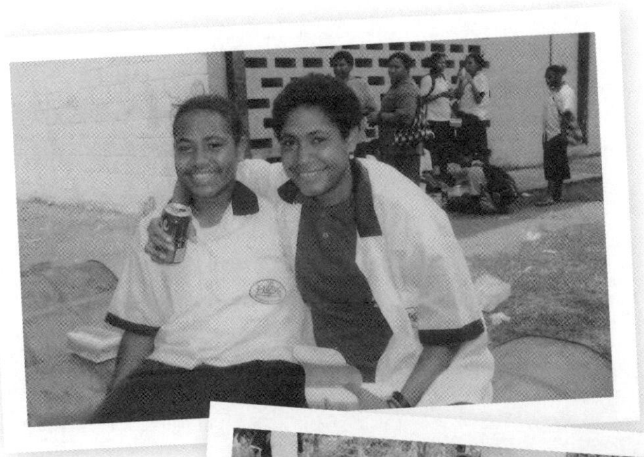

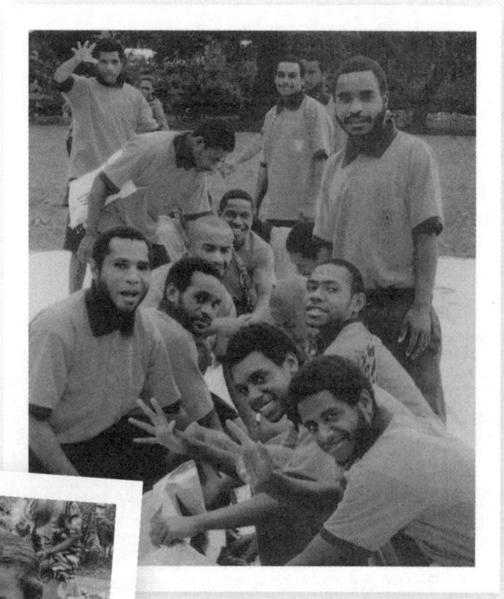

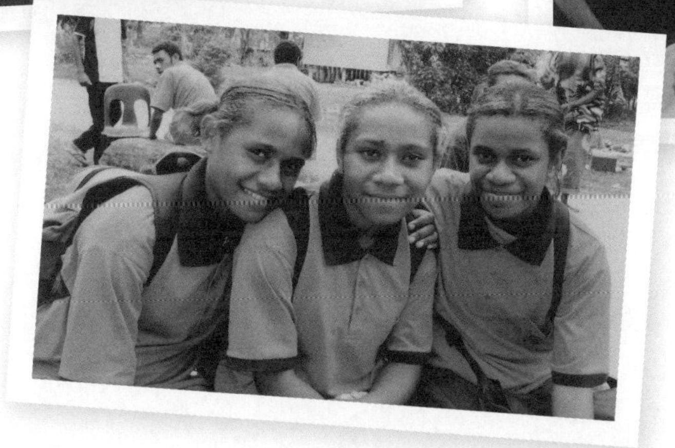

Being able to form strong and positive relationships is vital for the health of young women and men. Successfully managing relationships with others is something which will be valuable throughout their entire lives.

This book explores the challenges of the relationships young people will experience as they develop into adults. It explains the behaviours and personal skills that young people can use to build strong personal, social and professional relationships.

Chapter 1 Who am I?

Understanding who you are is a key part of forming healthy relationships. Knowing your values, your personality, your likes and dislikes helps you find a positive place among your friends and in the community.

What makes you who you are?

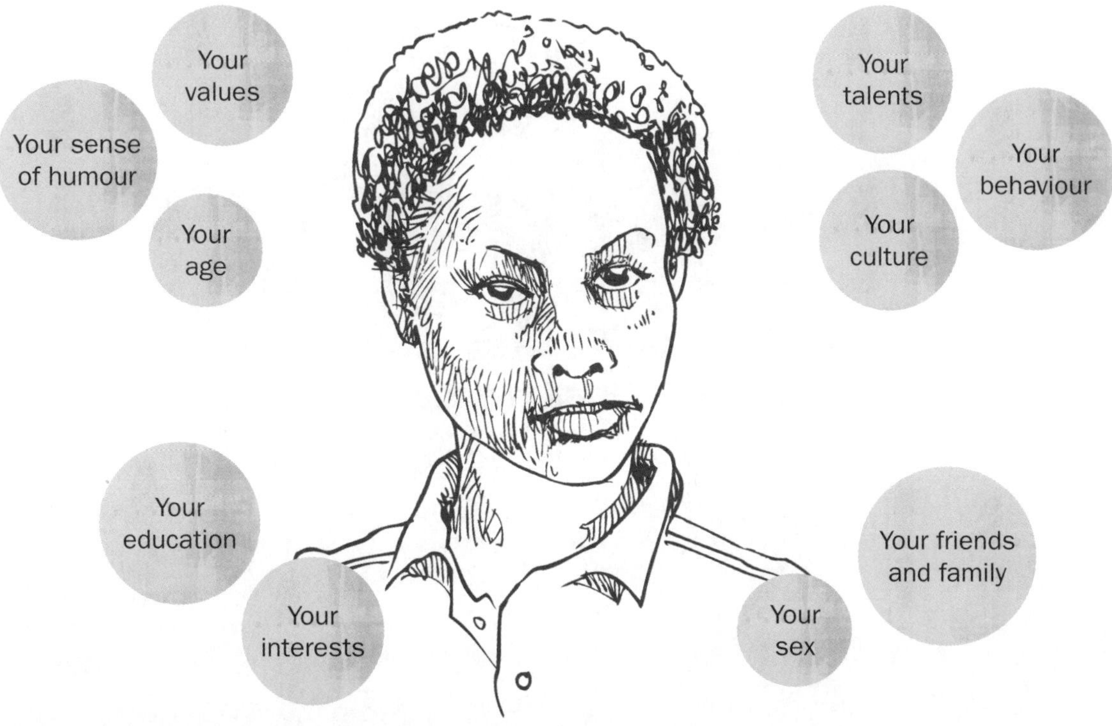

Your identity has been shaped by many factors as you have grown up. As a young child, these influences would have come largely from your family and community. As you got older, your friends, school and the media would play a larger role. Your individual personality will continue to develop and change throughout your life.

The relationships you form with other people will also develop and change throughout your life. They will depend on your personality and how you behave.

Activity 1•1 WHO AM I?

Reflect on these questions.

1 How do I feel about myself:
- my talents
- my values
- my interests
- my behaviour
- my culture
- my education
- my strengths
- my achievements?

2 How do I feel about other people:
- my parents
- my brothers and sisters
- my fellow students
- my friends
- my community?

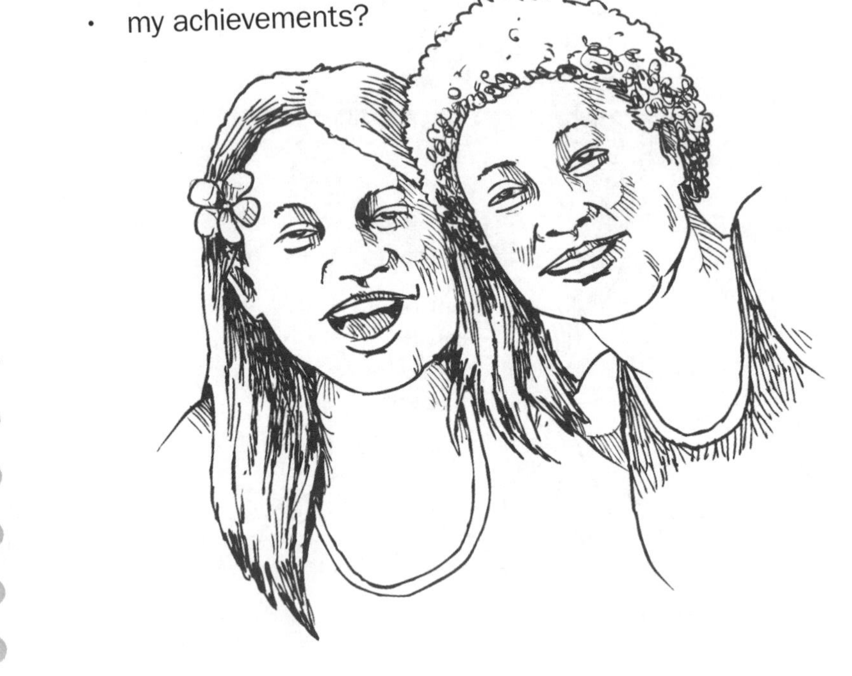

How you feel about yourself is called **self esteem**. Self esteem can affect how well you form and manage relationships. If you have high self esteem you are positive and realistic about your values, talents and achievements. You treat yourself with respect and deal with problems maturely. People with low self esteem think negatively about themselves.

Other people can affect your self esteem. Being bullied can harm your self esteem and self confidence. Being praised or complimented improves how you feel about yourself.

It may take many years for a young person to fully develop emotionally. Along the way, many young people will experience high self esteem and low self esteem. They may experience high self esteem one day and low self esteem the next day. This can depend on the people they are with, the setting they are in and how they are feeling about themselves at the time.

Being able to see yourself as other people do is one way of being able to form better relationships. How you behave towards others is very important.

If you are a caring, honest and supportive person you are more likely to have caring, honest and supportive relationships.

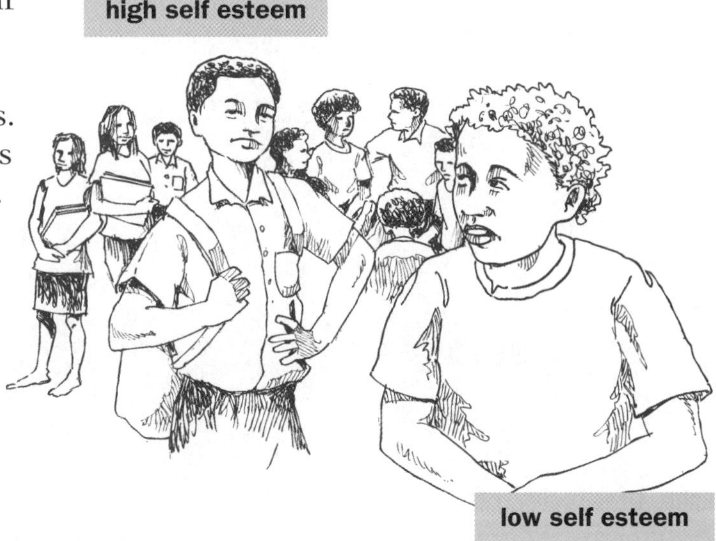

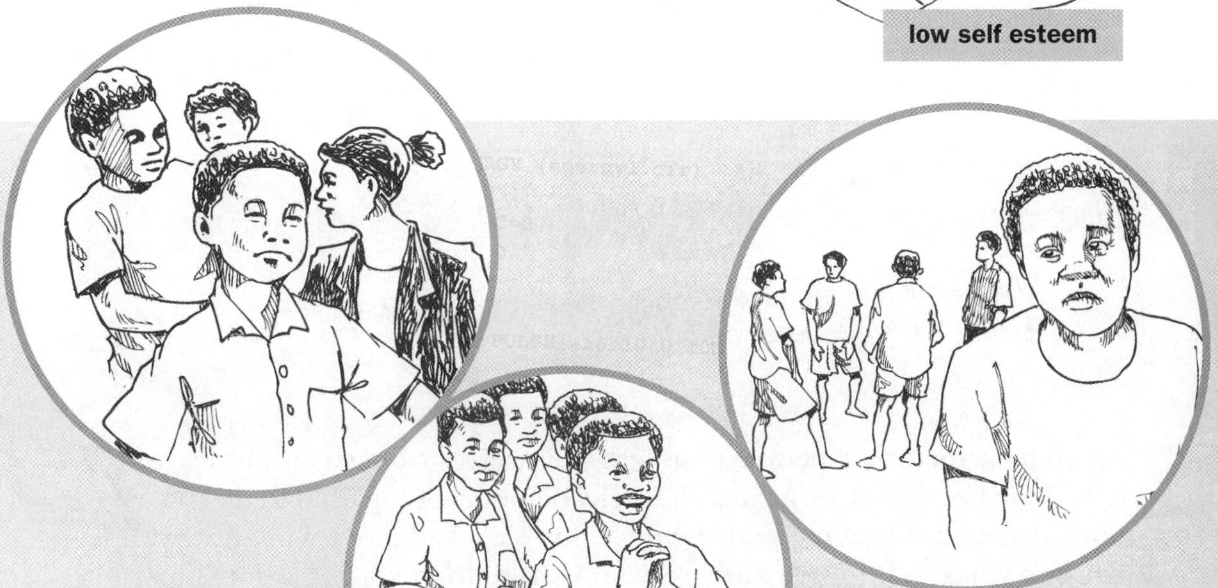

Activity 1·2 WHAT DO PEOPLE THINK ABOUT ME?

Ask two people you trust to describe you and then compare this to your answers in Activity 1.1.

	How ______ describes me	How ______ describes me	How I described myself
talents			
values			
interests			
behaviour			
strengths			
achievements			
how I treat others			
areas I need to improve on			

What similarities and differences do you notice? Why do you think they see you differently?

It can be difficult for people to assess themselves honestly and to admit that their behaviour or attitudes might be poor. Being able to do this is a powerful skill. Knowing your own weaknesses and flaws will allow you to develop ways to improve and grow and strengthen your relationships.

We all have many different kinds of relationships. The main thing that is the same in all those relationships is *you*. Behaviours and attitudes that build healthy relationships must start from your own personality and behaviour.

Chapter 2 My relationships

Everyone has many different kinds of relationships. These might include relationships between:

- parents and children
- brothers and sisters
- wantoks
- friends
- boyfriend and girlfriend
- husband and wife
- teacher and students
- patient and health worker
- employer and employee
- players on a team
- pastor and church members
- community members.

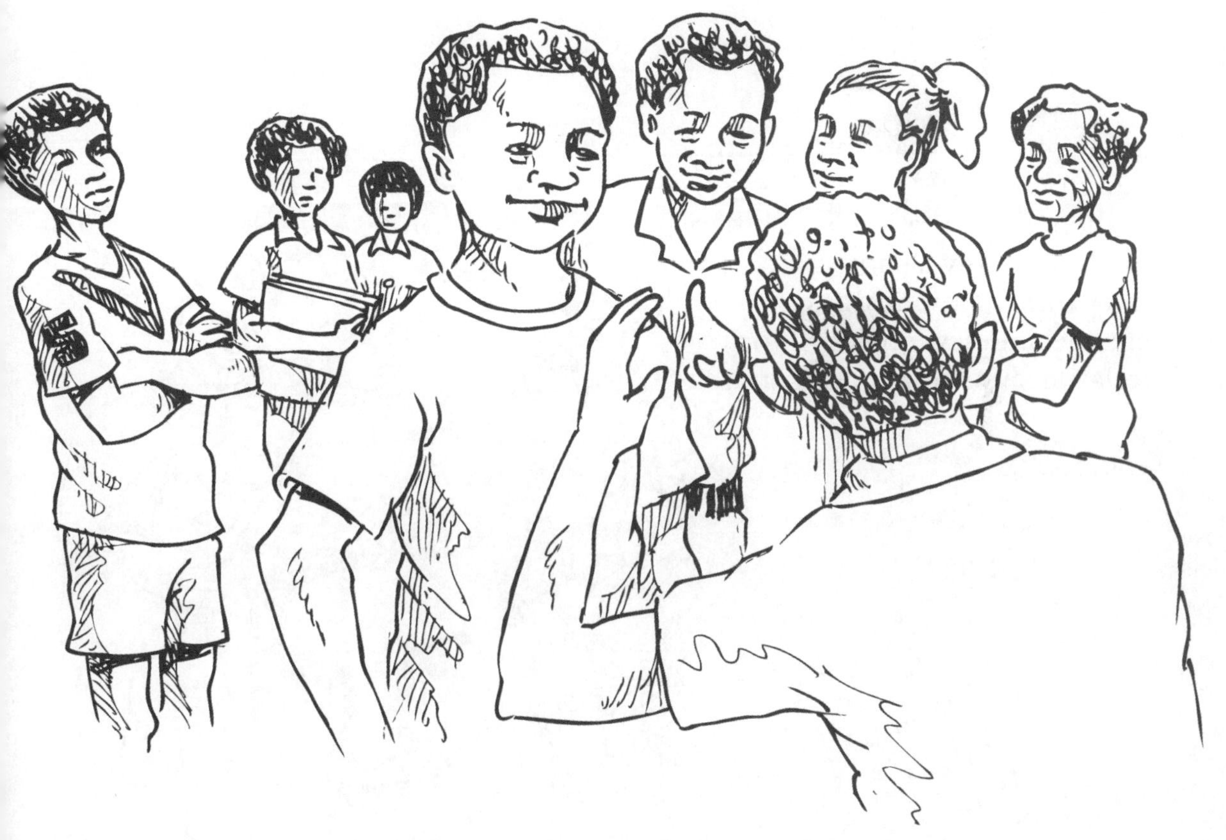

Activity 2·1 BRAINSTORM

1. Work with a group of friends and list other relationships from within your community, school and family.
2. Now underline the relationships which you have now. For example,
   - Employer — Employee
   - Sports captain — Player
   - Politician — Voter
3. Finally, discuss each relationship.
   - Why is this type of relationship important?
   - When will you start to have this kind of relationship?
   - Which relationships are the most important to you now?
   - Which relationships might be more important to you in the future?

Some of these relationships are more important than others. Some of them last a lifetime and others might last only a short time. Over time relationships can change and new ones will form. Relationships might even end.

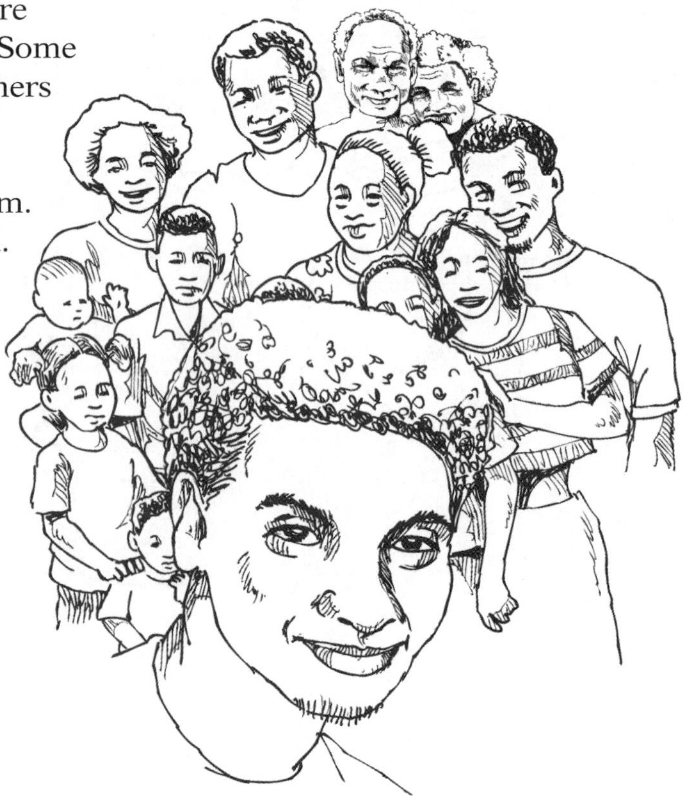

Relationship pyramids

Look at this pyramid of important relationships. Most people have many acquaintances but very few (or even just one) intimate partner.

Intimate partners are people you are having a romantic or sexual relationship with. You would share your most intimate thoughts, ideas and feelings with this person and trust them with important personal possessions and ideas. You might share a home and plan for the future together.

Close friends and family are people you have a deep relationship with. You might hug them. You would share personal ideas and feelings with them. Best friends would fall into this group.

Friends and extended family are people you see regularly and who you would shake hands with and talk to. You would spend time doing things together and would meet for special occasions and visits.

School and work colleagues are people you see regularly during the day. You have a formal working relationship with them.

Acquaintances are people you might see around in your community. They might be people in the market or shops. You would say hello to them and discuss only general topics.

Activity 2·2 WHO IS IN MY RELATIONSHIP PYRAMID?

- Complete a blank pyramid for your relationships. Enter the names of people in the right level of the pyramid.
- Do you think there are any people who would put you into a different category?
- Compare your pyramid with your friends' pyramids. How are your pyramids similar? How are they different?

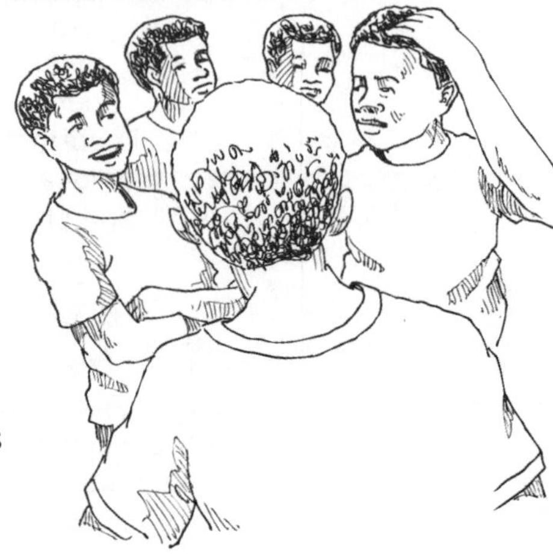

As we get older, our relationships change. During **puberty** we start to feel sexually attracted to others. Most people will eventually marry. Friends might move away and family members might die. An acquaintance could later become a close friend.

Sometimes it is difficult to balance the needs of different relationships. Most students will have many friends, some close friends, parents, siblings and teachers all making different demands on their time and energy. It helps to think about which are the most important relationships for you and why.

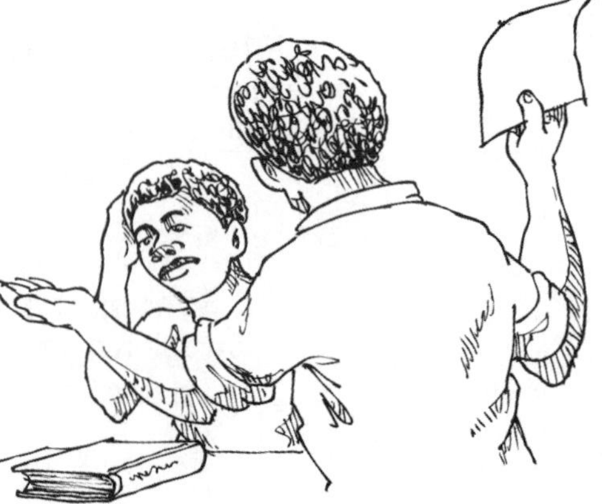

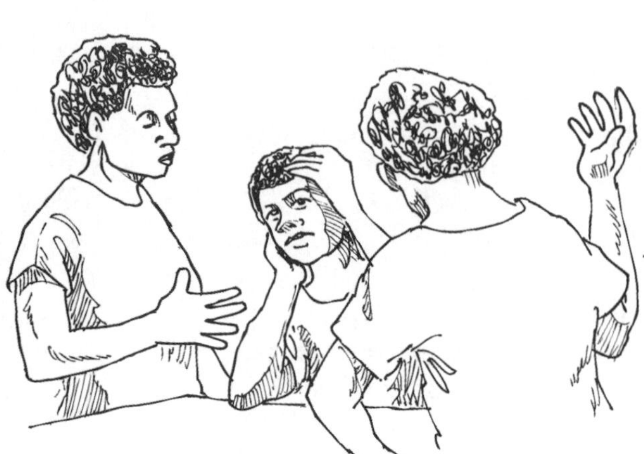

Activity 2.3 WHICH RELATIONSHIPS DO I VALUE THE MOST?

Look again at the pyramid of people in Activity 2.2.

1 Which are your five most important relationships? Why?

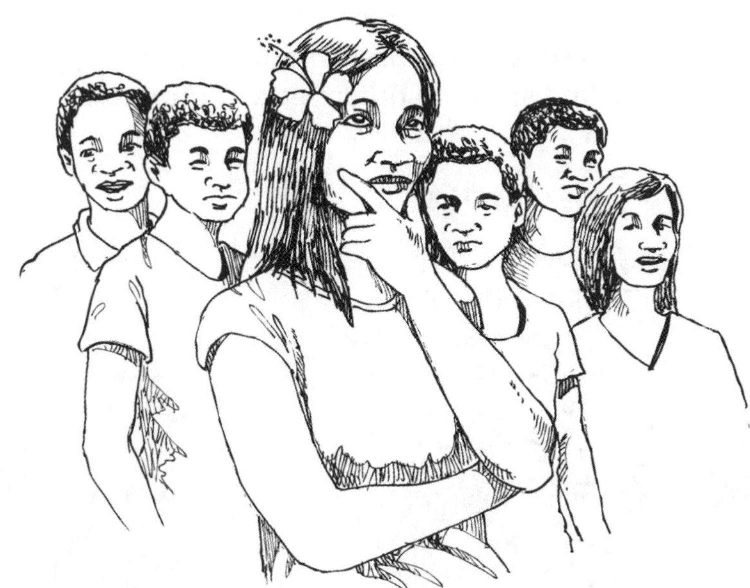

	My most important relationships	What makes them important
1		
2		
3		
4		
5		

2 Have the relationships that are most important to you changed in the last year?

3 Do you expect any of these relationships to change in the next three years? Why?

Chapter 3 Behaviours for healthy relationships

There are many ways we can strengthen our relationships with others. The way we behave and speak to others is very important.

Honest praise and compliments
I like the way you helped your little brother this morning. Well done.
Standing up for your rights and the rights of others
It is not fair or Christian to say that about her. I think you should apologise.
Listening and supporting
You seem angry this morning. What's up?

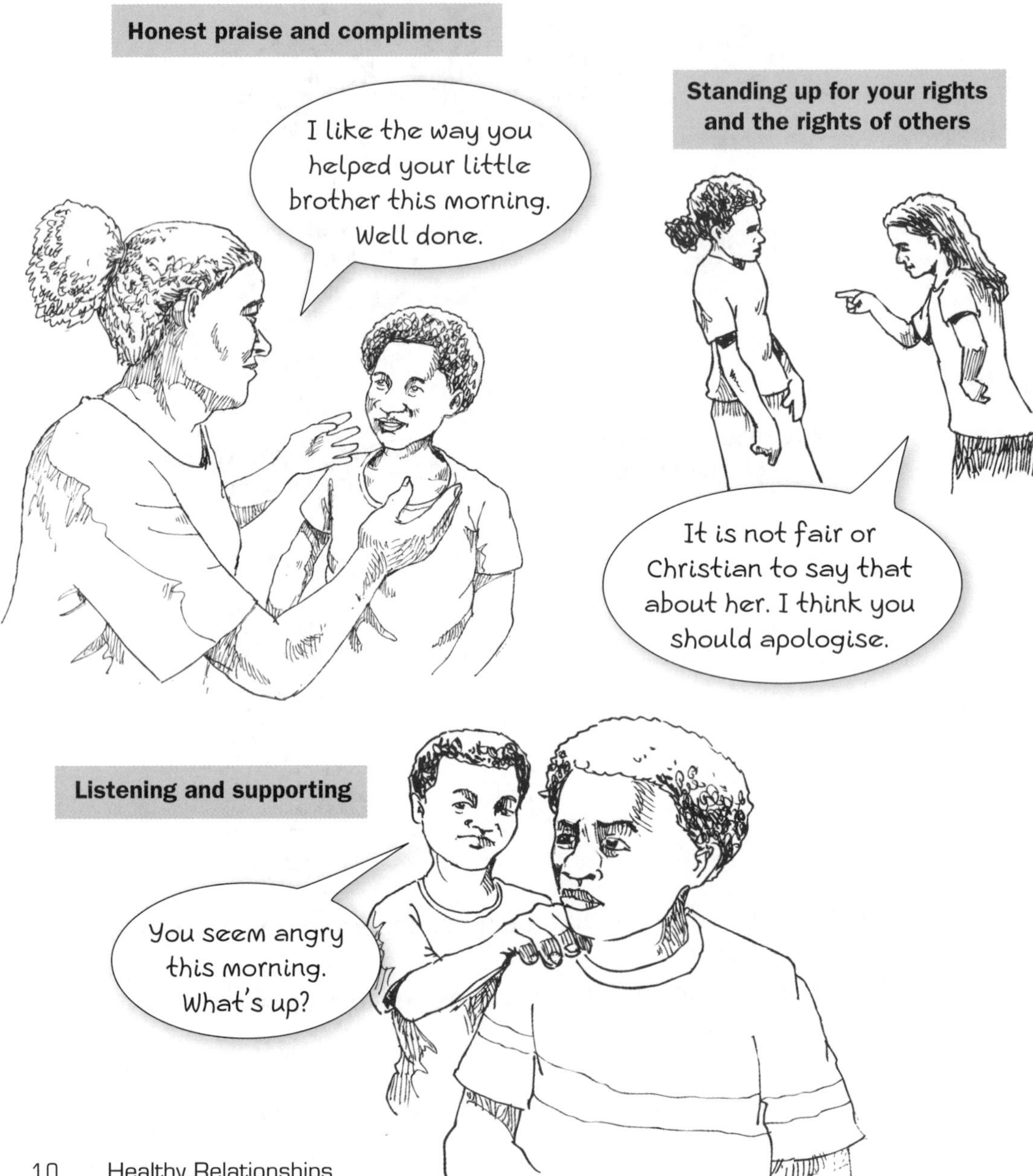

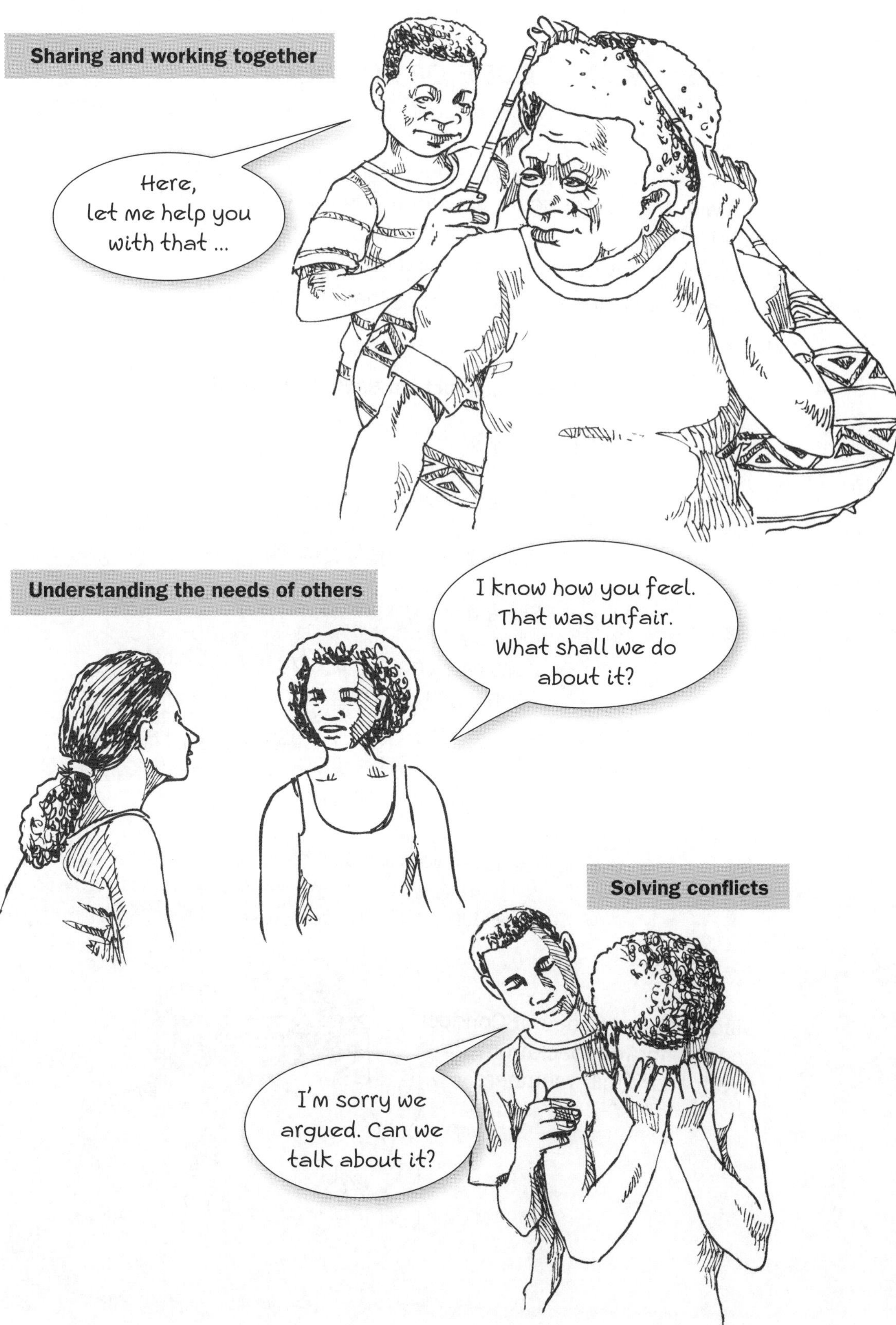
Sharing and working together
Here,
let me help you
with that ...
Understanding the needs of others
I know how you feel.
That was unfair.
What shall we do
about it?
Solving conflicts
I'm sorry we
argued. Can we
talk about it?

Activity 3.1 CODE OF CONDUCT

Choose at least one type of relationship from Chapter 2 and work with a group of peers to write a Code of Conduct for that relationship.

- Which behaviours help that relationship?
- Which behaviours might damage that relationship?

For example:

Code of Conduct between brothers and sisters

1. Be polite.
2. Respect each other's privacy.
3. Respect each other's property.
4. Share your toys, games and books if asked nicely.
5. If you have an argument, try to solve it before going to your parents.
6. Help each other with homework if asked nicely.
7. Share the chores fairly.
8. Be fair in your games.
9. Have fun.

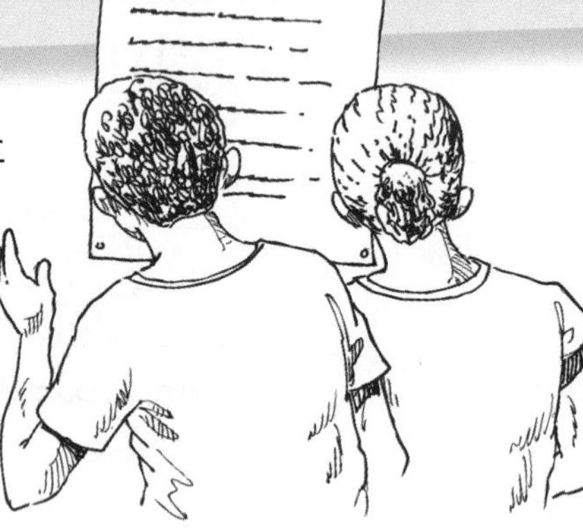

Display these Codes of Conduct and ask for feedback from peers and family members.

Rights and responsibilities in relationships

People have both rights and responsibilities in all relationships. For example:

Rights

All people have the right to:

- speak and be heard
- safety
- fairness
- health.

Responsibilities

All people have the responsibility to:

- respect the rights of others
- think for themselves
- take responsibility for their decisions and actions
- be honest and helpful.

Activity 3.2 RELATIONSHIP RIGHTS AND RESPONSIBILITIES

Look again at your Code of Conduct you wrote in Activity 3.1.

What are the rights and responsibilities for each of the people in your chosen relationship? For example:

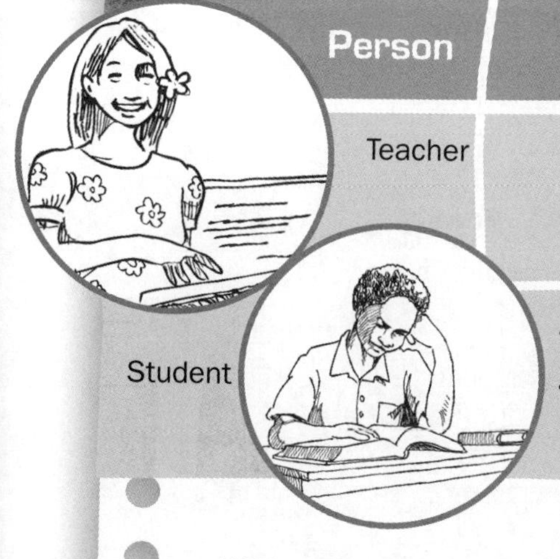

Person	Rights	Responsibilities
Teacher	• to have a safe work place • to be treated politely by students	• to be accurate, honest and constructive • to treat students fairly
Student	• to be safe at school • to receive a good quality education	• to work hard • to speak to the teacher politely

With a friend, discuss these two questions.

1 Are there any differences between the rights and responsibilities of the two people in the relationship? Why?

2 Are there any universal rights and responsibilities which every relationship needs?

Respect

One universal rule for healthy relationships is to show respect for the other person's rights, values, culture and views. This does not mean you have to agree with them or do what they say! You can politely disagree and you can try to persuade them to change their mind. In some situations you might just have to agree to disagree.

Activity 3.3 HOW DO I EARN RESPECT?

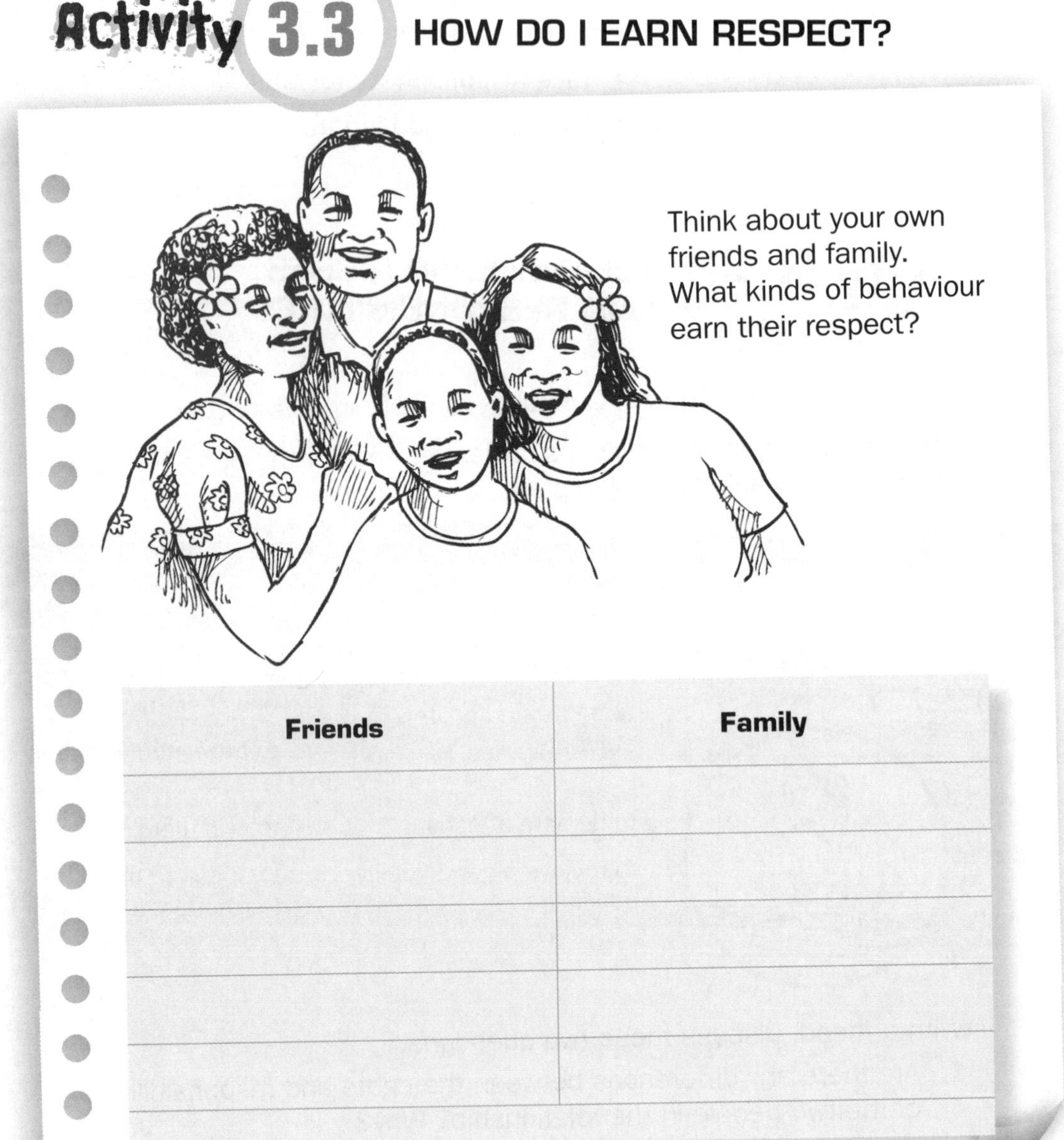

Think about your own friends and family. What kinds of behaviour earn their respect?

Friends	Family

In PNG, there are some situations in which it is expected that an individual be treated with respect because of their age, sex or position in the community.

Activity 3.4 WHEN RESPECT IS GIVEN BUT NOT EARNED

- Are there any situations where respecting someone without question could cause problems? Discuss these with a group of friends.
- Is it always right to respect and follow the opinions of others? For example, respecting the opinion of a tribal leader who wants to fight another village.

 Unhealthy relationships

The most common cause of a relationship becoming unhealthy is when one person in the relationship has too much power over the other person. This can be for many different reasons:

- cultural reasons
- traditional reasons
- social reasons
- family reasons
- educational reasons
- professional reasons.

When one person has too much power they can control or force the other person to make decisions or do certain activities. There are many relationships in which there is a difference in power. It is important that the difference in power is appropriate to the situation.

Type of Relationship	Healthy use of power	Unhealthy use of power
Teacher–student	Teacher asks student to stay after class so he can help him with his assignment	Teacher beats a student because he doesn't understand
Parent–child	Parent asks child to make her bed and keep her clothes tidy	Parent forces child to stay home from school to look after her siblings

Activity 3.5 APPROPRIATE AND INAPPROPRIATE POWER

- It is important to know the differences in power in relationships. If the power is misused it can be unhealthy and dangerous.
- Consider the different relationships from Chapter 2.
- Work with a group of peers to identify differences in power that might exist in these relationships. When is this healthy?
- When is this unhealthy?

Behaviours that promote healthy and unhealthy relationships

Positive behaviours

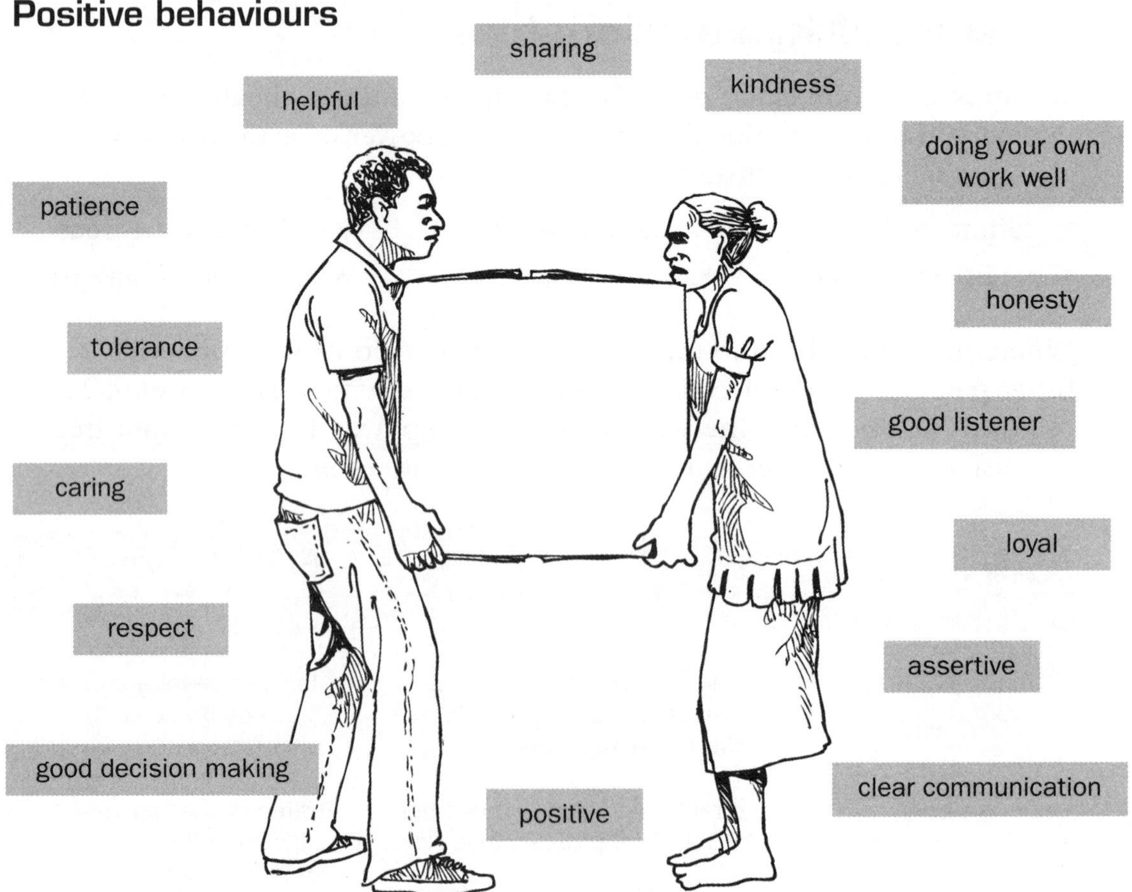

Negative behaviours

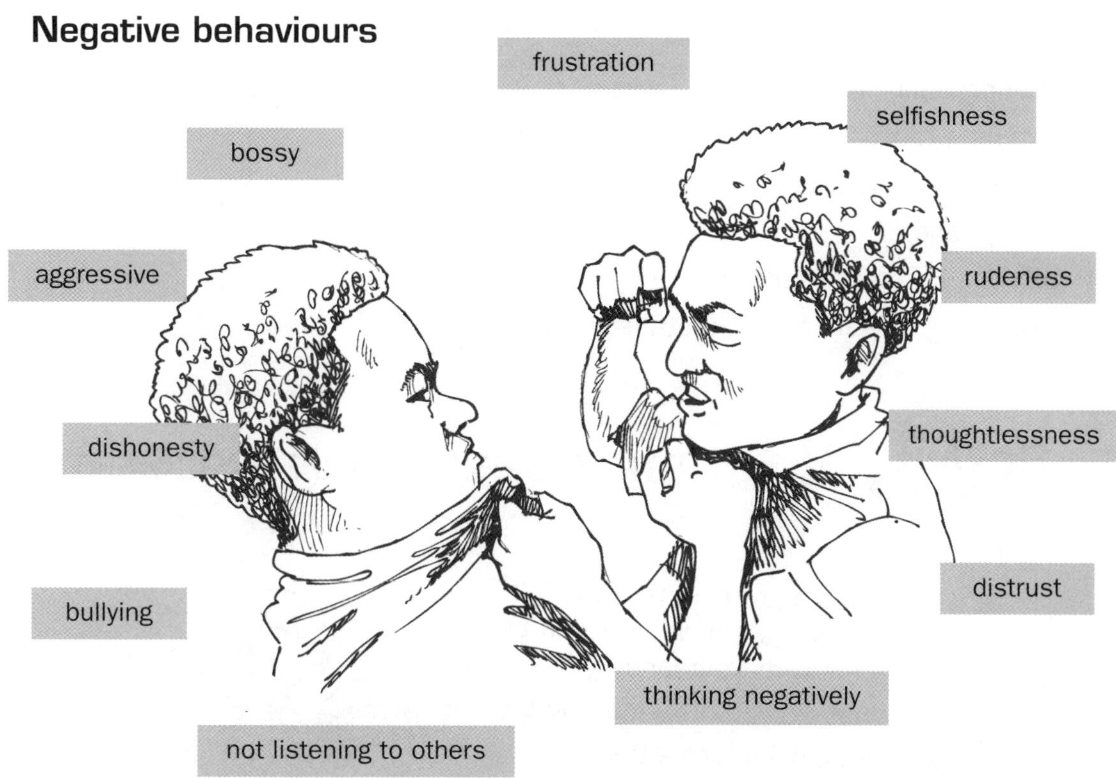

Conflict resolution

It is common for people to disagree about a certain issue, decision or action. If everyone was the same, life would be very boring. What is important is how people handle their difference of opinion.

Often, disagreements can be resolved through calm and controlled discussion and debate. In the worst situations, disagreements are resolved through violence and even war.

In PNG, the village court magistrate system helps to settle village disagreements without violence. This is a long-standing practice.

When arguments and disagreements happen it is important that they are resolved so that the relationships are not harmed. People use many different strategies for **conflict resolution**.

Some strategies to solve disagreements include:

- staying calm
- listening to what the other person is saying
- asking someone else in the family to help
- being honest
- offering different solutions
- respecting one another and other people's opinions.

Activity 3.6 STRATEGIES TO SOLVE ARGUMENTS

1 Work with a group of friends. Talk about a time when you were in an argument with someone.
   a What did you disagree about?
   b How did you solve the disagreement?
2 Compare the different stories.
   a What were some of the strategies people used to solve their disagreement? (For example, talking, learning, understanding, including a trusted adult, fighting.)
   b Which strategies were most successful?
3 Which strategies will you use in the future to solve disagreements?

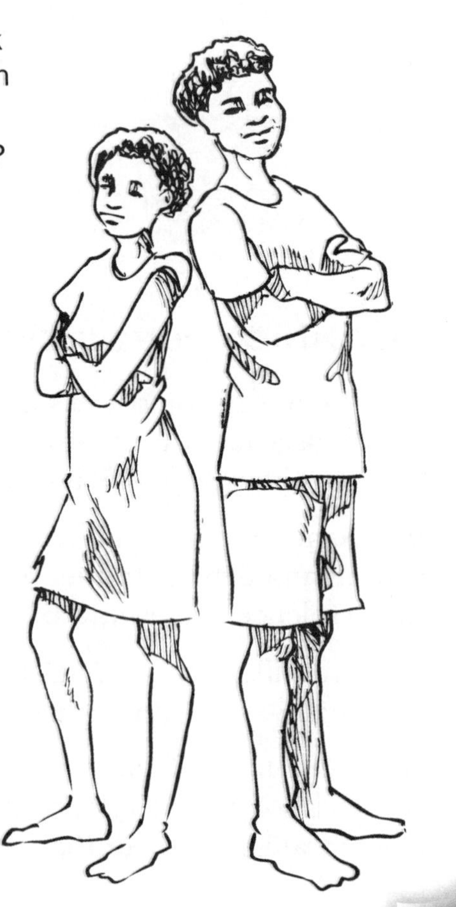

Chapter 4 Relationships with your family

In the Pacific, family groups are very important. There are many different kinds of families depending on your culture, religious beliefs and the individuals that make up the family.

Within a family group there might be many different types of relationships. People have different roles and responsibilities.

These roles and responsibilities can change over time. For example, as you get older you become more independent, and after puberty you might start a family of your own.

Families provide social, emotional and physical support for each other, especially for children.

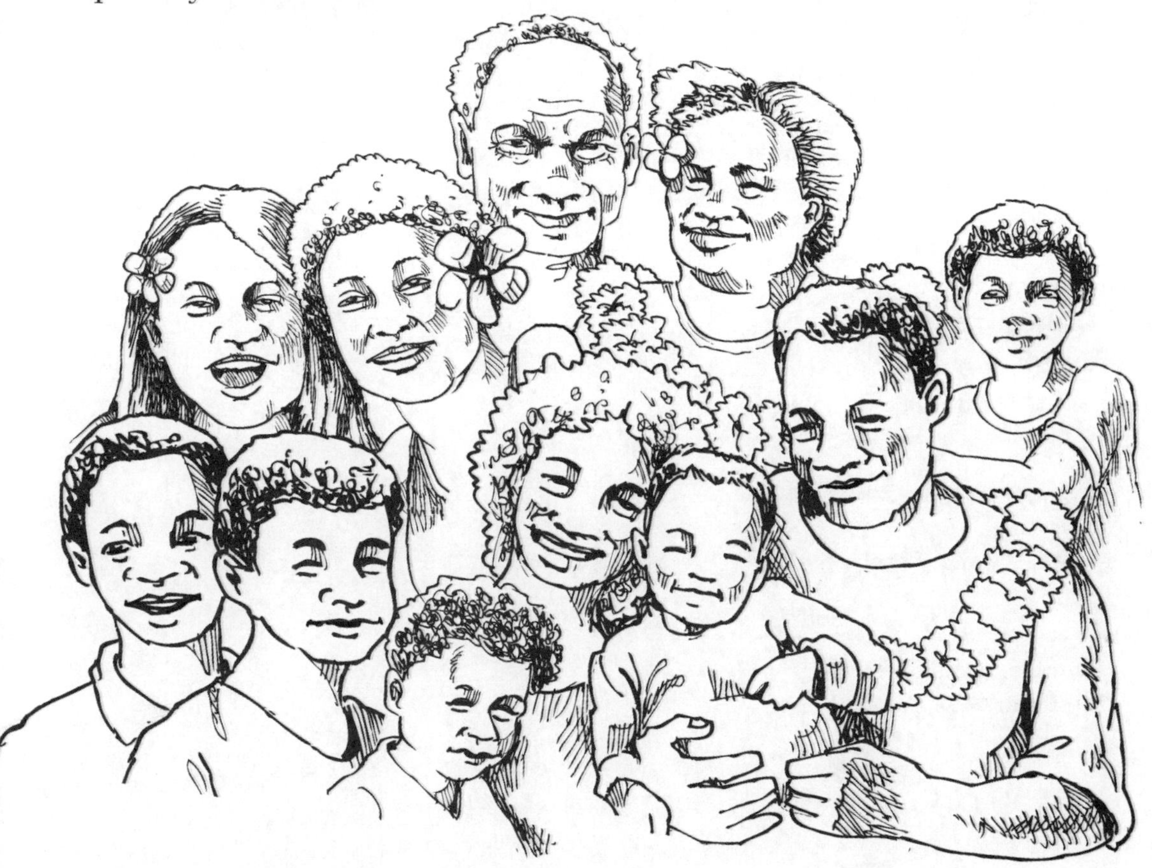

Activity 4.1 ROLES AND RESPONSIBILITIES IN YOUR FAMILY

In your own family, people may have different roles and responsibilities. Draw a picture of each member of your family and complete the table for each. Remember each family will be different.

For example:

Family member	Roles	Responsibilities
Mother/ wife	Working with father to provide food, shelter, safety and education	Love and care for children and love and care for husband
Father/ husband		
Children		
Adolescents		
Grandparents		
Aunties, uncles and wantoks		

Different types of families

There are many different types of family structures in Pacific cultures. In your community and clan you will see many of these. Although each structure is different, each relies on strong and loving relationships, which are crucial for good health and happiness.

These are some of the different family types found in the Pacific.

Extended family

- Several generations live together, sometimes in one house.
- Aunties and uncles visit frequently.
- There may be more than one set of parents in the family.

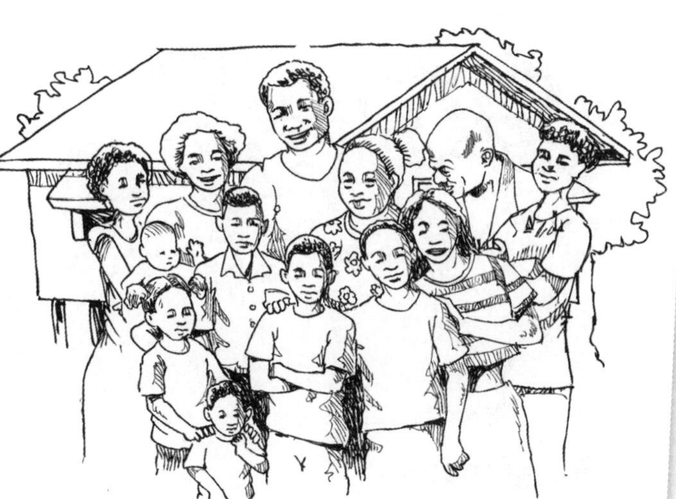

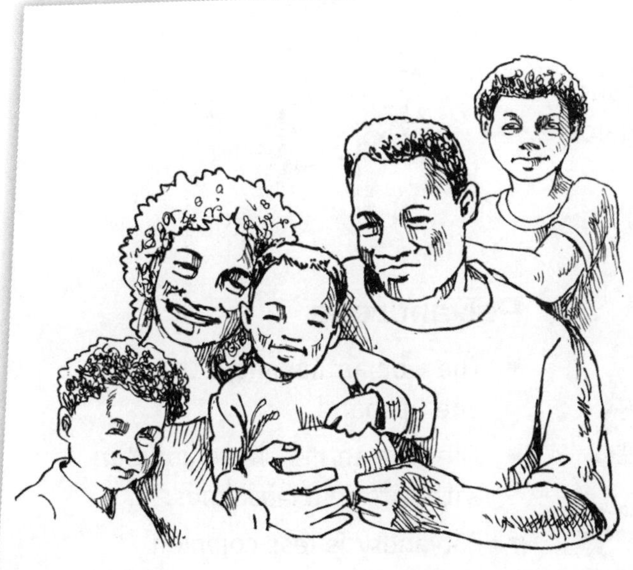

Nuclear family

- A nuclear family consists of parents and children only.
- Other relatives might visit.
- The family might live a long way from other family members.

Single parent

- There is only one parent in charge of the family due to separation, divorce, death, or one parent working away from home.
- The parent may have extended family or grandparents helping.

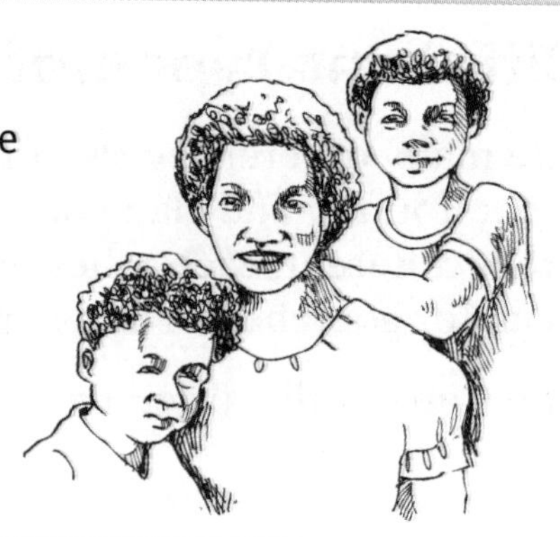

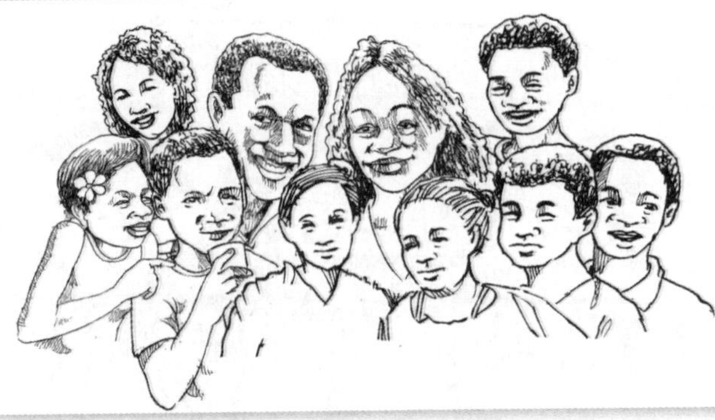

Blended

- One or both parents have children from past relationships.
- Sometimes the children have a wide range of ages.

Polygamous

- The man has more than one wife.
- The man may have children with different wives.
- The family may share one house, or have separate houses and gardens.

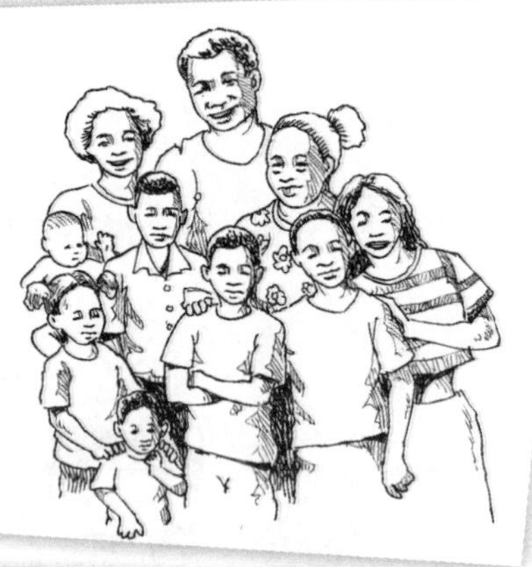

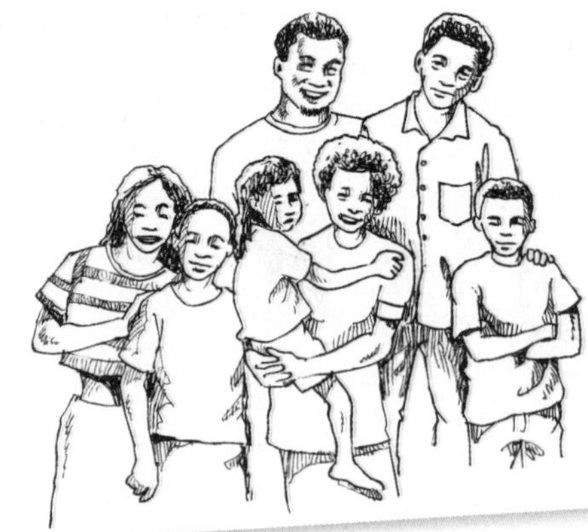

Polyandrous

- The woman has more than one husband.
- The woman may have children with different husbands.
- Polyandry is less common than polygamy.

It is important to remember that family structures can change over time. New children may be born, family members may leave home, or people may re-marry.

These changes can be difficult and you can read more about them in Chapter 12.

Activity 4.2 FAMILY TYPE SURVEY

Design and conduct a survey to answer this question:

Which family types are common among your fellow students and in your community?

1 Were you surprised by what you found out?
2 Why were some family types more common than others?

Remember

Be polite and respect confidentiality. There are many different types of families. There may be sensitive reasons for why your friends' families are structured in a particular way. Respect the rights and privacy of your friends.

Although the ideal family structure would be to have two parents who love, respect and care for each other, many families function well with only one parent. Similarly, just because parents have been married in church does not mean they would be able to raise children properly.

The most important thing for families is that the relationships within them are healthy and loving. Healthy families are built on healthy relationships.

Healthy family relationships require:

- love
- kindness
- respect
- trust
- sharing
- working together
- solving problems peacefully
- listening
- being patient
- helping everyone to stay healthy and have an education
- supporting family members through hard times.

Dealing with problems in a family

Every family will have problems in its relationships from time to time. This is normal. Within your culture and your family you might have special ways of dealing with any conflicts.

The best way to solve relationship problems is to prevent them from happening in the first place.

How are these people preventing problems?

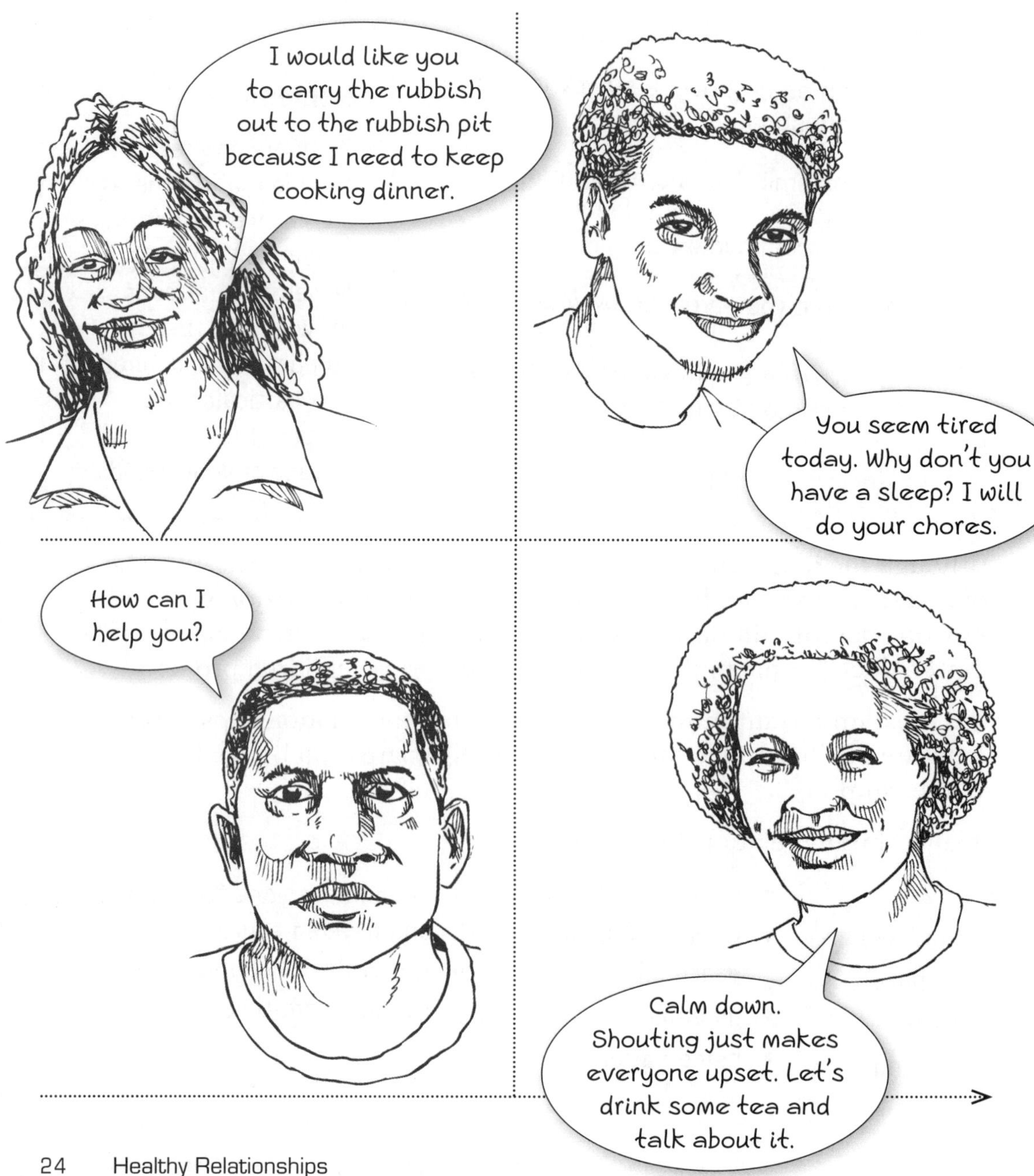

I don't think you should wear those clothes because you could get into trouble at the dance.

I love you, but I don't want to do that. What else can we do?

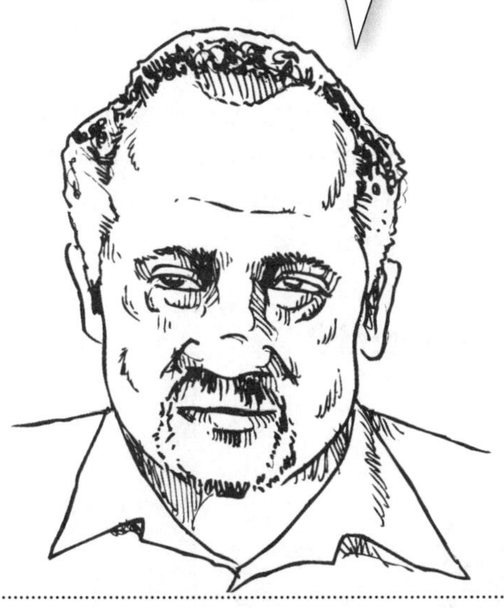

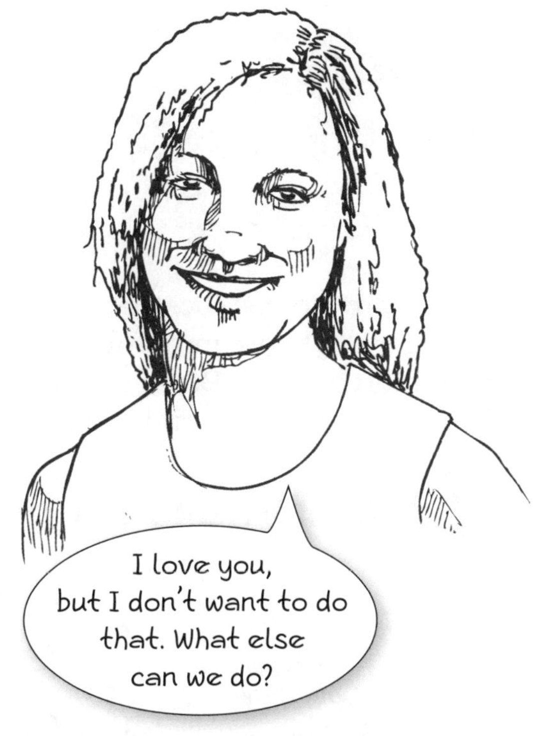

Activity 4.3 WHAT CAUSES ARGUMENTS IN FAMILIES?

With a group of peers, discuss these questions.

1. What causes arguments in your families?
2. Which family members are more likely to have arguments?
3. How are these arguments resolved? Can you use any of the strategies presented in Chapter 3 under Conflict Resolution?

Chapter 5 Friendships

As you grow older, the relationships that you have with friends become stronger and more important. Building and keeping good friendships is an important skill. Being a good friend and choosing good friends will bring you happiness and support throughout your life.

What makes a good friend?

keeps promises
sense of humour
intelligent
understanding
respects my opinions
good listener
keeps secrets
doesn't push me to do things I don't want to
dependable
forgiving
honest
similar interests
supportive

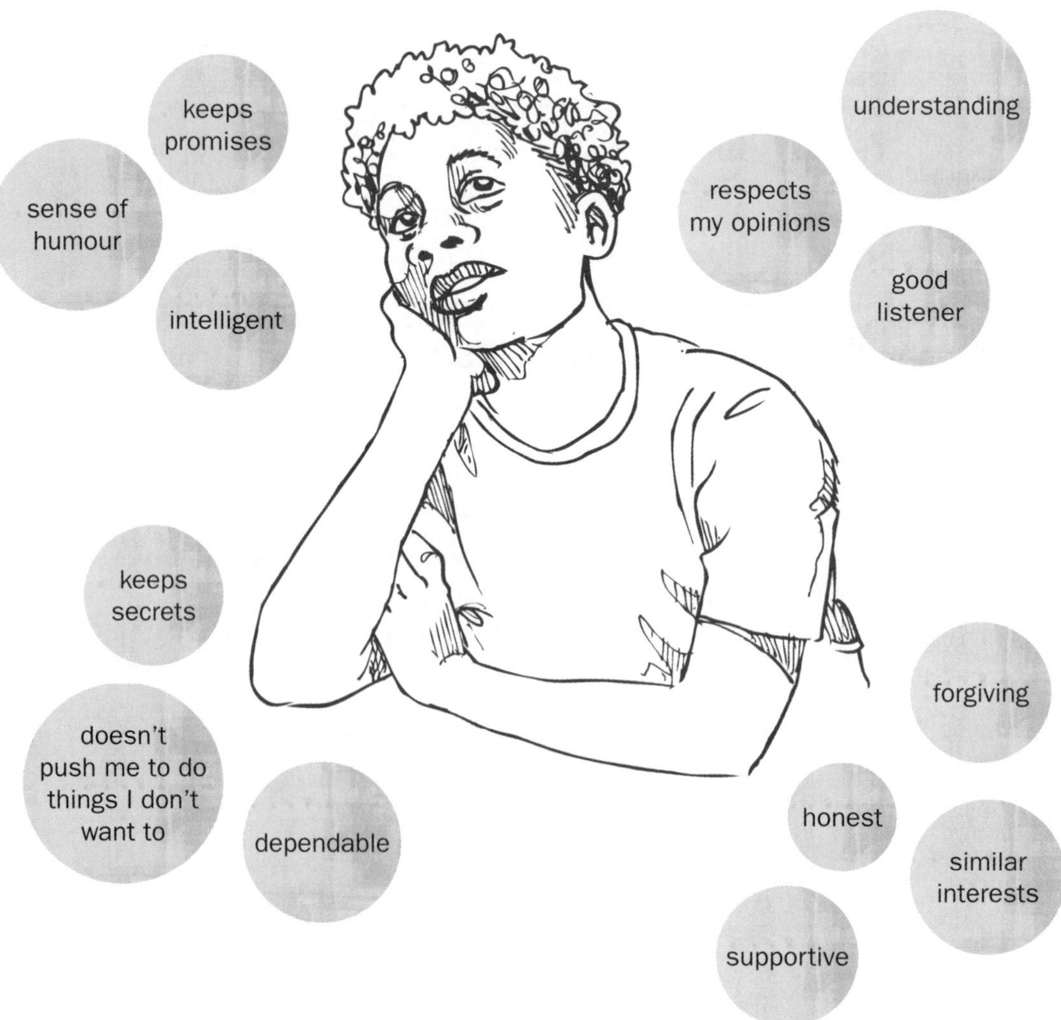

Activity 5.1 QUALITIES I LOOK FOR IN MY FRIENDS

Think of people you consider your close friends. What qualities do they have that make them a good friend? Are there qualities that are not presented in the pictures below?

Fill in the table below for three of your friends. What qualities do you look for most in your friends?

	Quality	**Quality**	**Quality**	**Quality**
Friend 1				
Friend 2				
Friend 3				

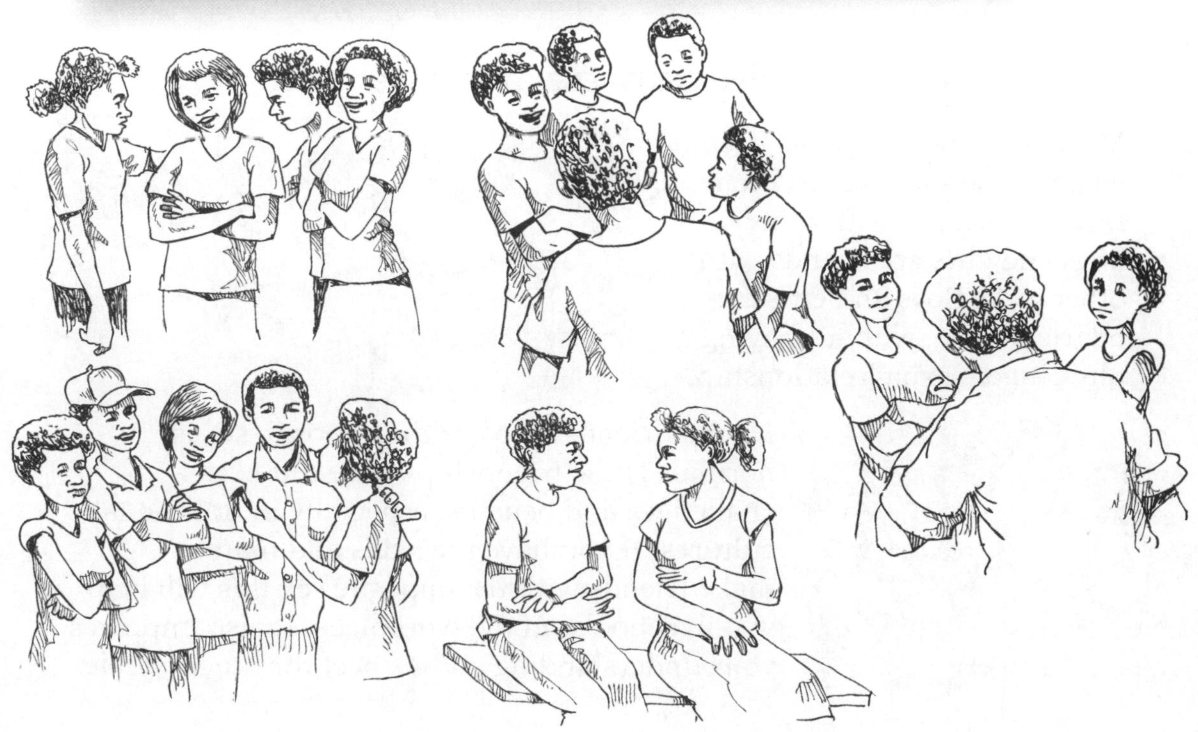

Activity 5.2 ARE YOU A GOOD FRIEND?

Keeping good friends requires you to be a good friend.

1 Answer each question below from your friends' perspective. Would your friends say that you:

• are a good listener?	**Yes**	**No**	**Sometimes**
• can keep secrets?	**Yes**	**No**	**Sometimes**
• respect their privacy?	**Yes**	**No**	**Sometimes**
• pressure them into doing things?	**Yes**	**No**	**Sometimes**
• are honest?	**Yes**	**No**	**Sometimes**
• are supportive and understanding?	**Yes**	**No**	**Sometimes**
• get mad easily?	**Yes**	**No**	**Sometimes**
• are dependable?	**Yes**	**No**	**Sometimes**
• are helpful?	**Yes**	**No**	**Sometimes**
• are generous?	**Yes**	**No**	**Sometimes**
• are patient?	**Yes**	**No**	**Sometimes**

2 Consider your answers. What does this tell you about the kind of friend you are?

Boys and girls can be friends too!

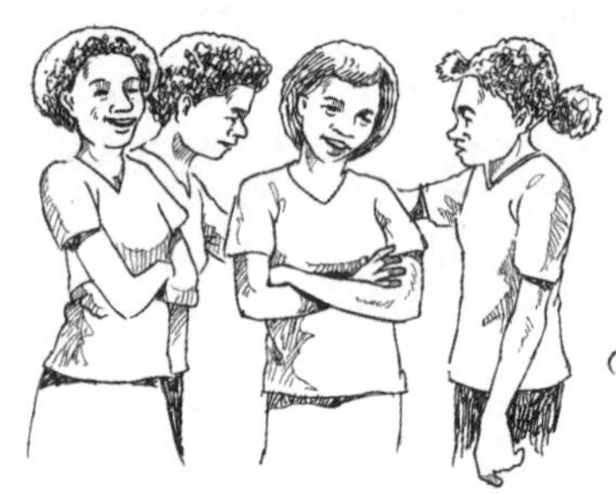

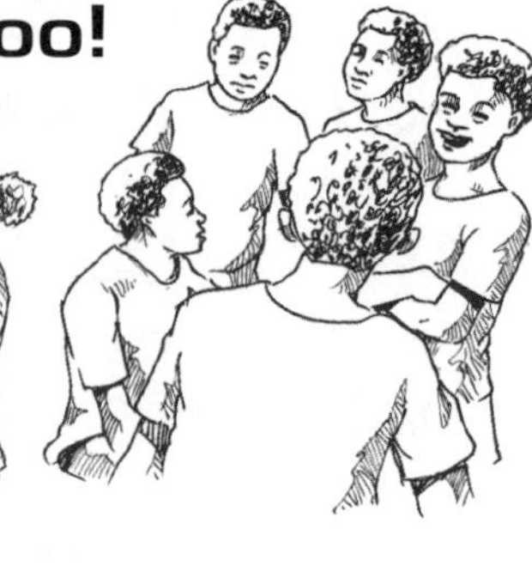

Most boys and girls have friends who are the same sex as them. Boys are friends with other boys and girls are friends with other girls. Boys and girls can be friends too, without having a physical or sexual relationship.

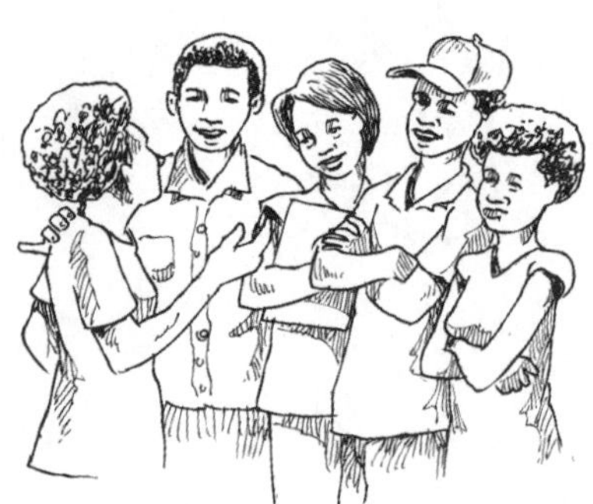

Having friends who are the opposite sex is normal. These friendships have different challenges and benefits, especially in traditional cultures. If you have the skills and maturity to make friends with the opposite sex this will help you in school and the workplace. It also improves your understanding and respect for other people.

Activity 5.3 BOYS WHO ARE FRIENDS AND GIRLS WHO ARE FRIENDS

Girls and boys experience different benefits and challenges from their friendships. Girls who have friendships with boys might experience different challenges than boys who have friendships with girls.

Fill in the table below. Discuss your ideas with your friends.

If you are a girl

	Friendships with other girls	Friendships with boys
Benefits		
Challenges		

If you are a boy

	Friendships with other boys	Friendships with girls
Benefits		
Challenges		

Traditionally, **adolescent** boys and girls do not spend a lot of time together. Cultures and traditions are changing, though, and you may develop friendships with people of the opposite sex at school, at church or in your community. Some older people may find this difficult, but being able to make friends with the opposite sex is important in the workplace and in school. It is important to respect their opinion and to help them understand the importance of friendships between boys and girls.

When you make friends with someone of the opposite sex, it is important that they have the same qualities, values and interests that you would look for in a friend of the same sex.

Groups of friends

Most people have a group of friends. This can be a small group or a large group. Your group of friends may include people who are very similar to one another, or people who are very different from one another. Your friendship with each of your friends will be different too. The different activities you choose to do with different friends will depend on your friends' values, qualities and interests.

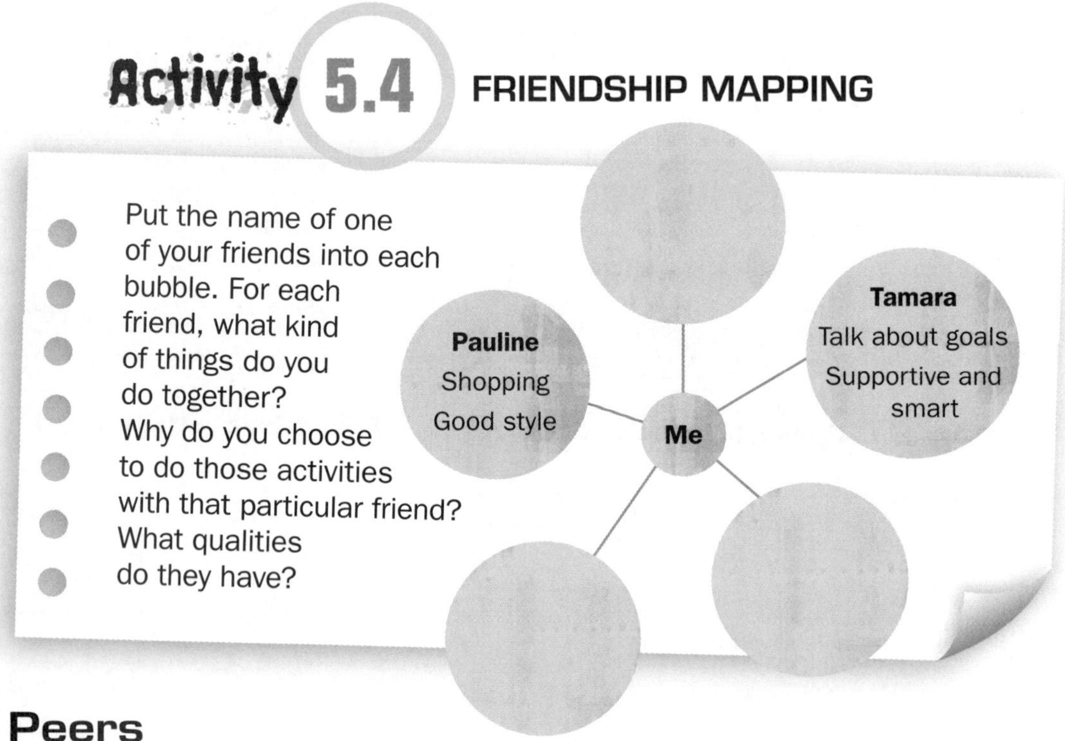

Peers

Someone who is your **peer** has things in common with you such as age, gender, interests or life experiences. Young people like to feel accepted by their peers. A peer may be one of your friends or they may just be an acquaintance.

You may belong to several different peer groups: for example, classmates, sports team, youth group.

Activity 5.5 YOUR PEER GROUPS

List the different peer groups you belong to. Compare these with a friend. List friends who are also peers. List peers who you may not also consider to be a friend.

Disagreements

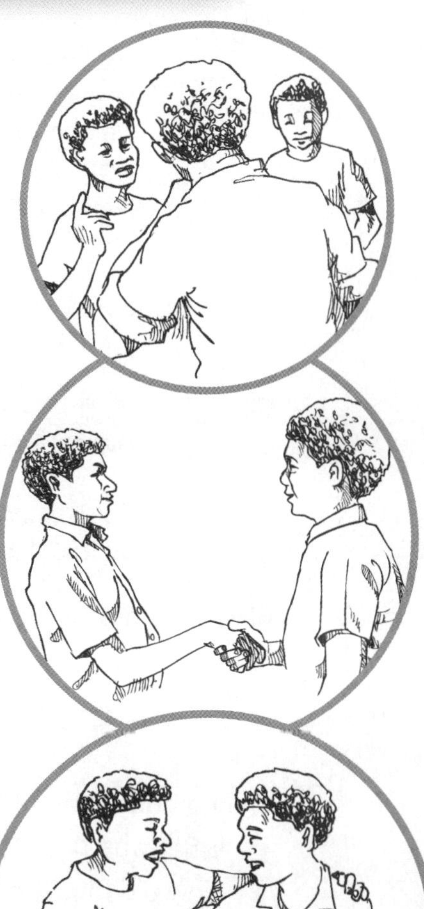

As with any relationship, there will be times when you don't agree with your friend or you have an argument. Building skills to handle problems or disagreements with your friends will help you to have long-lasting friendships.

Disagreements and problems in friendships can happen for many different reasons. When disagreements happen, people might feel hurt, upset or angry. Sometimes a person will not even realise that they have upset their friend, or what they have done to cause this.

If you have an argument or are upset by your friend it is important to do something about it. This is best done in a calm way. It is important to explain how you feel and why you feel this way.

Review the conflict resolution strategies that you developed in Activity 3.6. These may have included some of the following strategies:

- talking
- learning
- understanding
- including a trusted adult
- patience.

It is important to talk about problems as quickly as possible. You may feel uncomfortable doing this and it may be difficult, but it is very important. If you leave an argument for a long time, then it can become more serious. The situation can become confused and bad feelings can grow. The sooner you deal with the problem, the easier it will be to solve.

Case study: Tamara and Elly

Elly: Tamara, can I talk to you about something?

Tamara: Sure. What's up?

Elly: Tamara, I was really upset yesterday when you didn't meet me at the library. We were going to study for our test, but you didn't show up. I saw you later hanging out with your friends and this made me really angry and sad.

Tamara: Elly, I didn't mean to upset you. I'm sorry. One of my friends was sick in the morning and I needed to get her to the aid post.

Elly: Oh, I'm sorry for your friend. I hope that you're OK. Still, you could have called or texted me to let me know.

Tamara: Yeah, that would have been a good idea and would have stopped you from being upset. I'll try to do that next time.

Elly: Thanks. I'll do the same. I am glad that we could talk about this.

Think about how Tamara and Elly resolved their disagreement.

1. What was the argument about?
2. How did Elly feel?
3. How did Tamara respond to Elly saying she had upset her?
4. What strategy did Tamara and Elly agree to use to avoid this situation in the future?
5. What strategies can you use to resolve arguments with your friends?

Chapter 6 Relationships in school

School is an important place of support for young people. Building and maintaining good relationships will help you be happier and more successful.

Sometimes young people have problems with other people in their school. You need to know how to prevent or solve these problems and help others to improve their relationships.

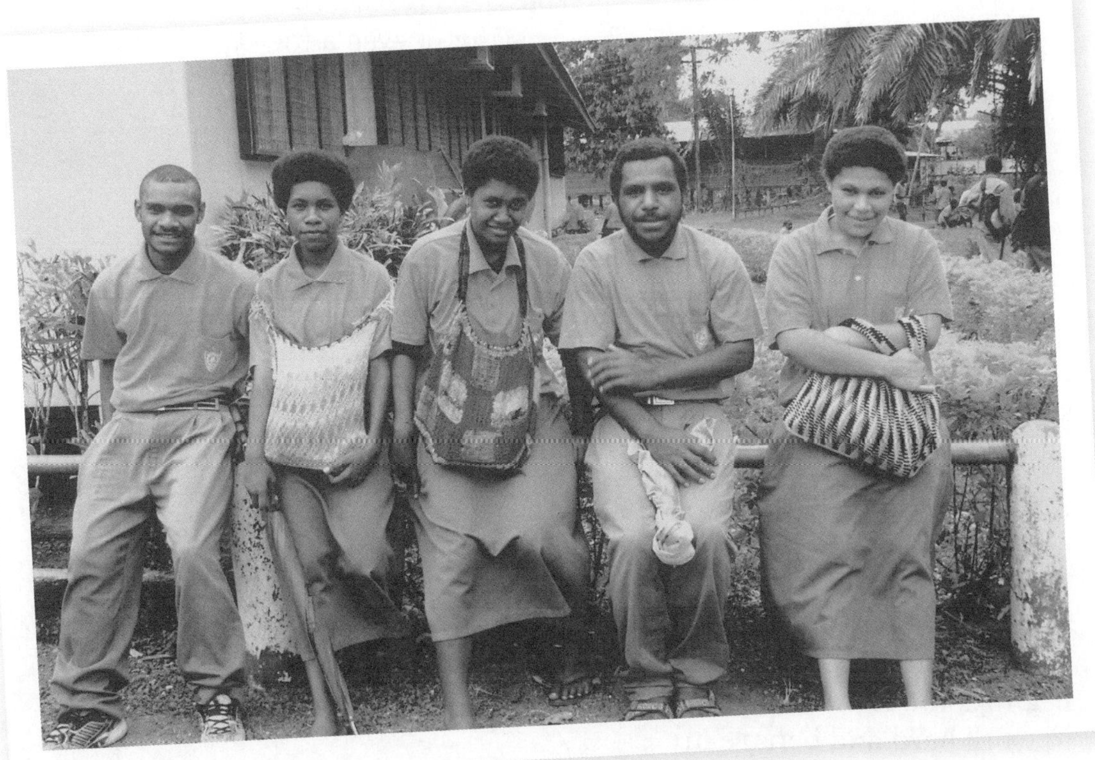

Activity 6.1 WHAT ARE THE KEY RELATIONSHIPS IN MY SCHOOL?

Draw a map showing the most important relationships you have in your school.

Choose a key to show which relationships are:

- professional
- friendship
- classmate
- other.

Think of how you will show how important each relationship is.

A professional relationship would be one between a student and a teacher. However, you might consider a teacher to be a mentor or even a friend.

Relationships between teachers and students

Teachers are an important part of growing up. Your relationship with your teacher is very important. You will need their support and help. They need you to work hard and behave well in the classroom.

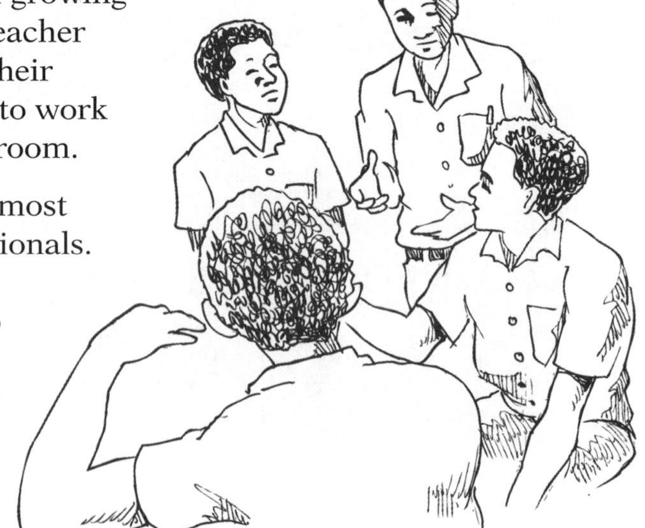

It is important to remember that most teachers are hardworking professionals. Teachers are paid to teach you. They have a responsibility to help you learn and keep you safe and healthy. You have a responsibility to work hard and behave in school. You have to do your job for them to be able to do theirs.

Activity 6.2 SELF REFLECTION: WHAT MAKES FOR A POSITIVE STUDENT–TEACHER RELATIONSHIP?

Think about the best and worst teachers you have had. Don't write down their names, but answer these questions about them.

My best teacher	My worst teacher
• How did he or she treat you? • What did he or she do to help you learn? • What did you have to do to make the relationship positive? • How did this teacher help you grow and develop as a person?	• How did he or she treat you? • Why didn't you learn well with that teacher? • How did you behave? • What could he or she have done to make the relationship better? • What could you have done to make the relationship better?

There are many ways to strengthen the relationship between teachers and students.

I will behave well.

I would like the students to be polite, hardworking and honest.

I will make sure I am at work on time and setting interesting and challenging tasks.

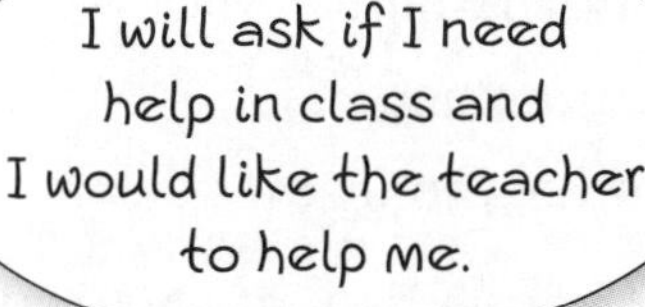

Activity 6.3 WHICH OTHER BEHAVIOURS IMPROVE RELATIONSHIPS BETWEEN TEACHERS AND STUDENTS?

With a small group of friends, draw a picture of a teacher and a student. Write more speech bubbles like the ones on the previous page to list the behaviours that would improve relationships between you and your teachers.

Start each sentence with either "I will ..." or "I would like him/her to ...".

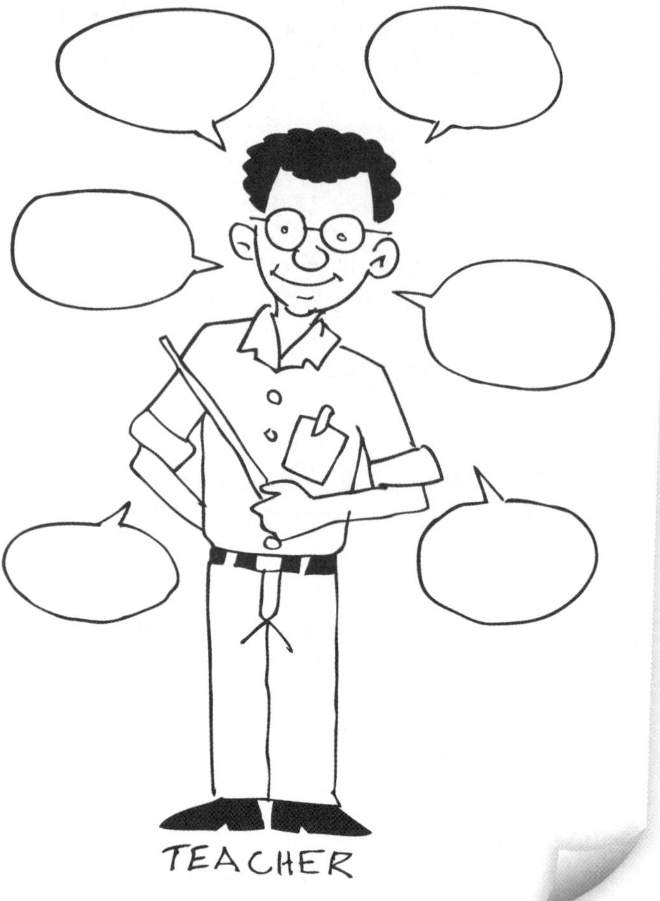

Most of these behaviours will be the same as the ones in your school or classroom rules. For example:

- be polite
- follow the instructions of the teacher
- be honest
- treat others fairly
- be hardworking
- help others to learn
- don't do anything that stops others from learning
- ask questions
- don't bully
- keep yourself and others safe and healthy.

These rules should also be followed by the teacher.

What to do if there is a problem between you and your teacher

As teachers are important people in your development, you should try to deal with any problems quickly. You can use your conflict resolution skills, ask others for help, speak to your parents or speak to another trusted teacher. Sometimes it is your own behaviour that is the cause of the conflict. A good friend could tell you if this is the case.

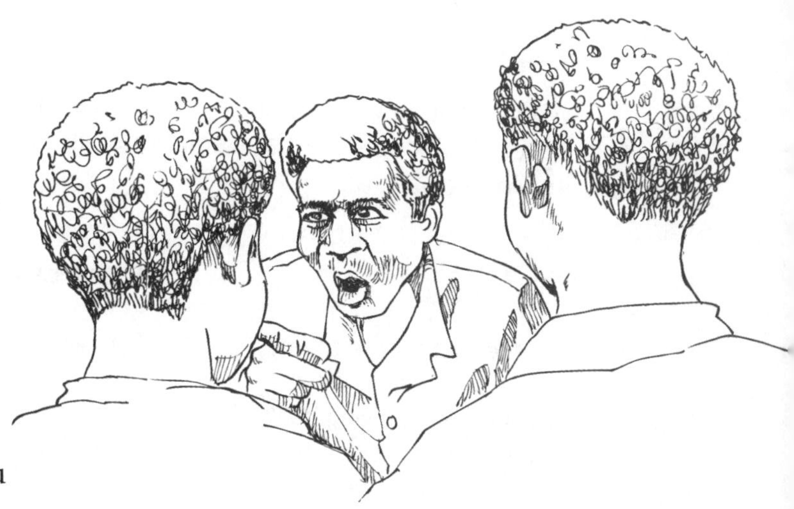

Dangerous relationships

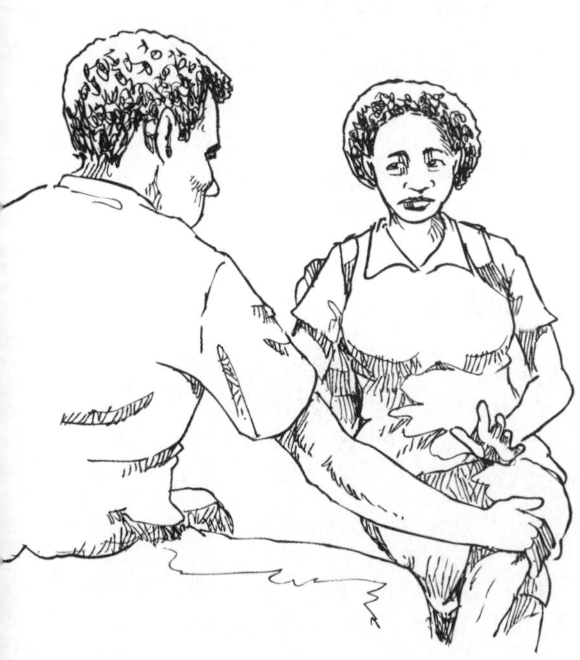

Most teachers are wonderful **role models** and hardworking professionals. However, if your teacher behaves badly or breaks the law, you must get help from a trusted adult, another respected teacher, the police or your parents. It is your right to be safe in school and teachers have a responsibility to ensure your safety in school.

It is an offence if a teacher:

- hits you
- bullies you
- punishes you in a cruel way
- treats you unfairly
- touches you sexually
- asks you to break the law
- asks for bribes.

Having sexual relationships with a student is illegal and the teacher will go to prison.

Activity 6.4 CLASSROOM CASE STUDIES

What would you do to solve these relationship problems in your school? Discuss the best solutions with a friend using your problem-solving strategies.

Case study 1

Every day your teacher seems to find some reason to punish you in class. You don't think you are behaving badly, but this has been going on since the start of term. You are starting to feel angry about it.

Case study 2

You are the teacher's favourite. You always get asked to answer questions first and the teacher keeps giving you special favours and praising you when you don't deserve it. It is starting to get embarrassing and your classmates are getting upset.

Case study 3

Yesterday when you were working you made a silly comment in class. The teacher told you off and you were rude back. You regret doing it now, but the teacher remains angry with you.

Case study 4

Your teacher keeps inviting you around to their house after school. They say that you can come around at any time. You don't think this is right.

Case study 5

Your teacher does not have good control over the class and you are finding it very hard to learn. The teacher seems very nervous. Your teacher has not taught this grade before.

Case study 6

Your teacher is flirting with you. You find your teacher attractive as well but you know this is not the right behaviour.

Case study 7

Most days your teacher is very late for class and last week they missed two whole days. The class is angry and wants to go on strike.

The National Behaviour Management Policy

To help improve behaviour in schools, the National Department of Education has written a National Behaviour Management Policy. Your school should have copies and it is also available on the Department's website: **www.education.gov.pg**

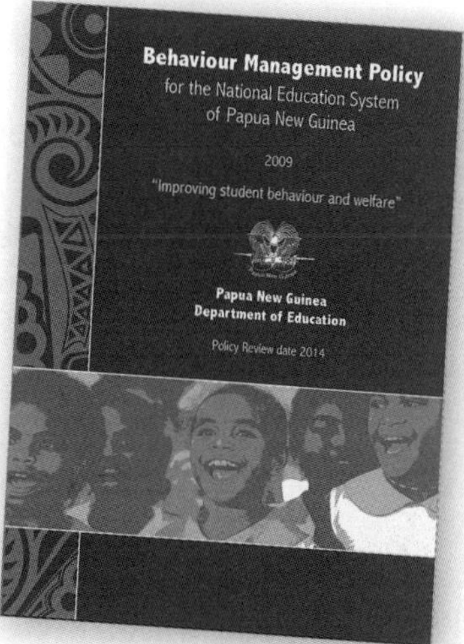

The Department of Education expects all students to:

1. Do their best in school.
2. Treat peers in a caring and friendly way regardless of their gender, sexuality, health, disability, religion, race or cultural background.
3. Solve problems and conflicts in a peaceful way.
4. Value school property and respect the properties of others.
5. Cooperate with fellow students, teachers and school authorities.
6. Actively contribute to decision making in the school and the Student Representative Council.
7. Try to be a good role model for others and encourage peers to behave well.
8. Be honest.
9. Report incidents of disruption, bullying, violence and any form of harassment.
10. Ask for help if they need it and help others.
11. Dress neatly in line with the school rules.
12. Come to school (don't truant) and attend lessons on time.

National Behaviour Management Policy, 2009, page 13

Activity 6.5 DISCUSSION ON THE NATIONAL BEHAVIOUR MANAGEMENT POLICY

1. Discuss the expectations of student behaviour from the National Behaviour Management Policy. Are they fair? Is there anything missing?
2. Compare these expectations with your own school rules and classroom rules. How are they different? How are they the same? Which rules are better?
3. Every school in PNG should have a Behaviour Management Policy that students, parents and teachers write together. Why is it important that everyone in the school is involved?
4. How do school rules improve relationships between teachers and students?
5. How do school rules improve relationships between students?

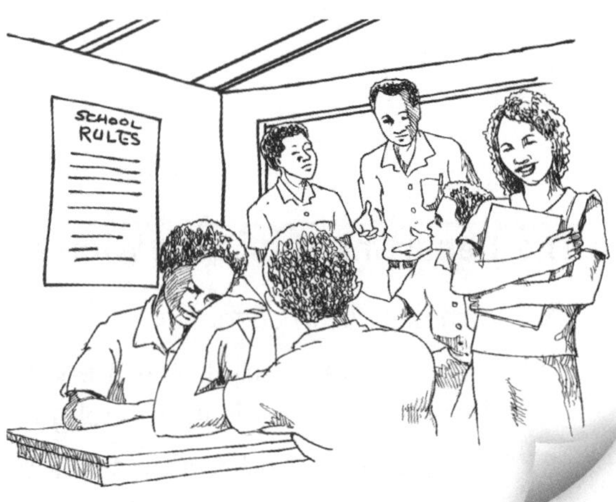

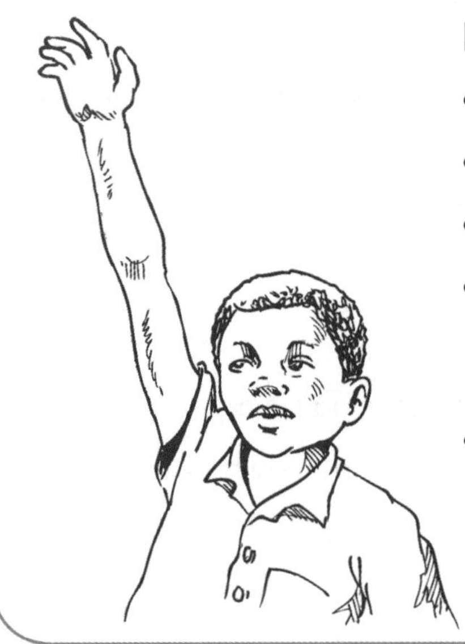

How to answer questions confidently

- Practise speaking loudly and clearly.
- Look at the teacher or class.
- Make notes before you answer.
- Practise what to say if you don't know the answer. ('I think it is ... but I am not sure.')
- Stand up and do not look at your desk when you are speaking.

Relationships between students

In school, you will have to work alongside many different students. Some might be older than you, some might be younger and some may come from different cultures and tribes.

Many of the good strategies for building and maintaining healthy relationships can be used in school. You also have the school rules which help students to behave well.

Relationships with your peers

You will work with your classmates every day, so it is important that you get on well with them. If someone is a bully you will need to do something about it. If someone is lonely or new in the class you should be welcoming and friendly.

Most importantly, the classroom should be a place for learning, and your behaviour should help that.

Working in groups

Working in groups can be a challenge. Here are some tips for good group work.

- Sit in a way that makes everyone feel part of the group.
- If you have a large group (more than five), split up into smaller teams.
- Make sure your group understands the task and ask your teacher if you do not.
- Elect a chairperson and a scribe (someone who makes notes).
- Remind everyone of the classroom rules before you start the task.
- Go around the table asking each person to give their views.
- Make sure that one person does not do all the talking.
- Ask questions to each group member.
- Divide up the tasks fairly.
- Keep an eye on the time.
- Say 'thank you' and 'well done' at the end of the task.

Activity 6.6 RIGHT OR WRONG?

1. Read this scenario from a PNG school. Discuss with friends what you would do next.
2. Now think about healthy relationships in your class. Write at least three other scenarios that could happen in school.
3. For each scenario, write at least three actions that would help to repair or maintain healthy relationships in the classroom.

> In your dormitory, your bunkmate keeps playing their radio late into the night. It keeps you awake. You tell them to stop but they ignore you …

Girls and boys, men and women

Most classes in PNG are mixed sex. This can make the relationships more challenging and interesting.

Traditionally, young men and young women did not mix very often. Nowadays they are expected to work together and learn together. This is good practice for modern life and the workplace.

Here are some ideas to help you work well with the opposite sex.

- Be confident and polite.
- Work in mixed groups.
- Make sure everyone is taking part in tasks.
- Offer to help.
- Encourage your friends to behave well around the opposite sex.
- Don't make sexist jokes or comments.
- Don't touch.

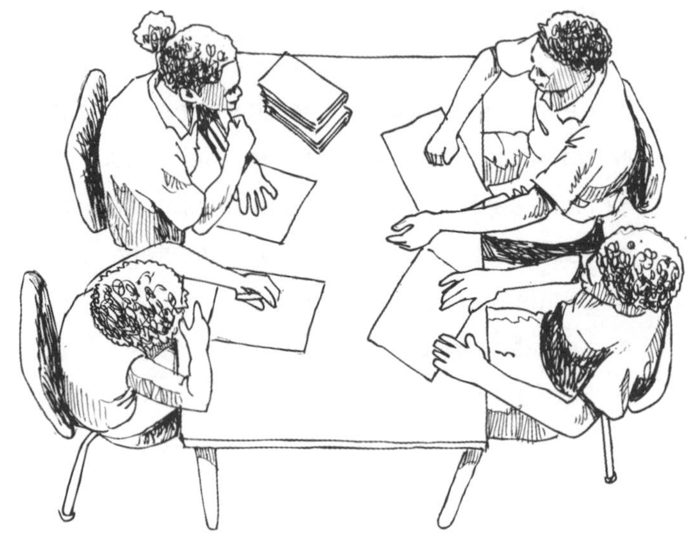

Relationships with younger students

There are many times that you will need to help younger students. It is a chance to be a positive role model. You should be someone who the younger students look up to and respect.

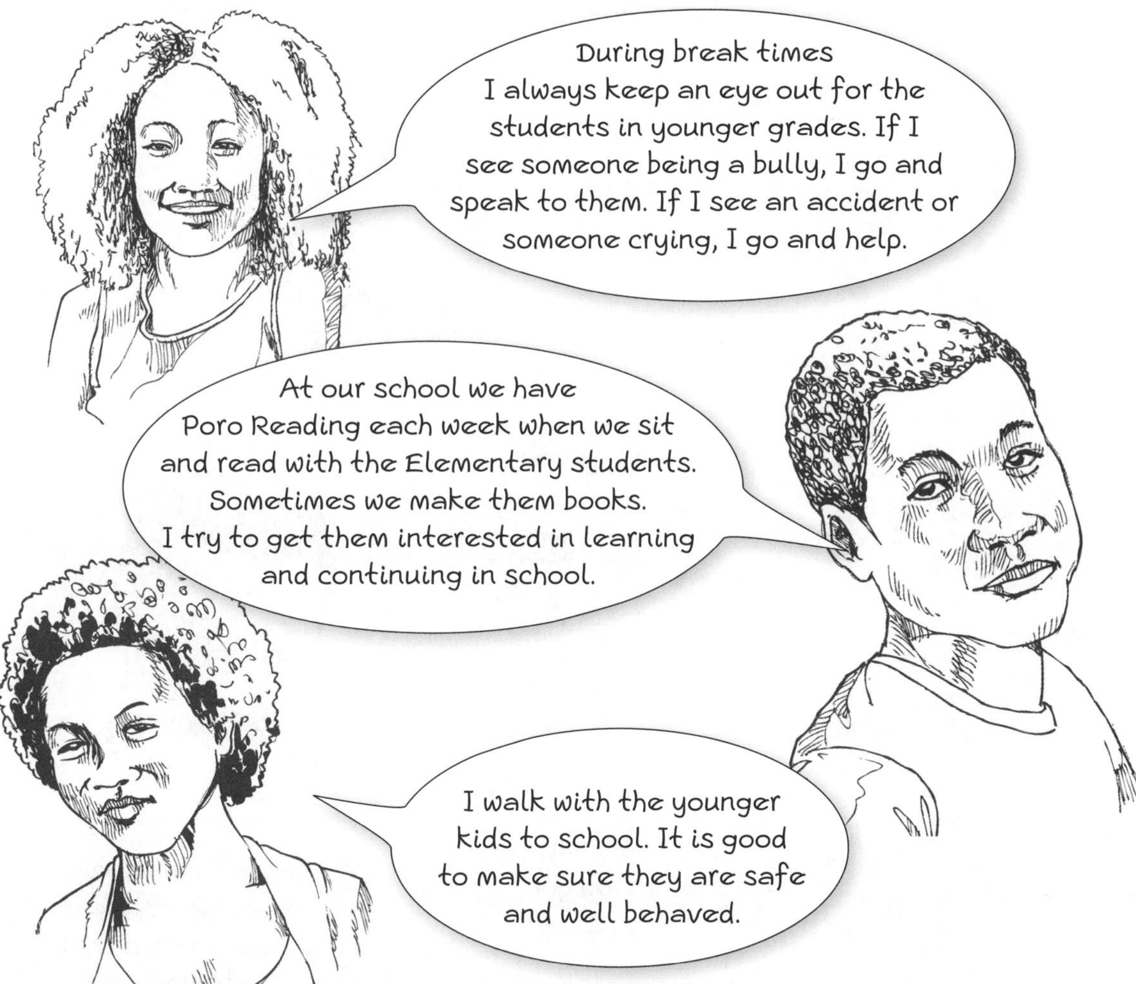

During break times I always keep an eye out for the students in younger grades. If I see someone being a bully, I go and speak to them. If I see an accident or someone crying, I go and help.
At our school we have Poro Reading each week when we sit and read with the Elementary students. Sometimes we make them books. I try to get them interested in learning and continuing in school.
I walk with the younger kids to school. It is good to make sure they are safe and well behaved.

Relationships with older students

Older students often seem to have a lot more experience and knowledge than you. Most older students will be friendly and helpful, but some might bully younger students.

You will probably have some friends and family members in older grades when you are in primary school, but when you start secondary school you might be the only person from your community at your new school. It is important that you avoid older students who could be a bad influence on you.

If you have problems with a relationship with an older student, speak to a trusted peer or respected teacher. Bullying is always wrong and it must be dealt with quickly. If you are bullied or you see bullying, do something about it.

These are some good phrases to practise:

Stop being nasty to me. You are bullying me.
Bullying is wrong. God is watching you.
Can I help?
If you try and bully me I will try and stop you.
Leave them alone. You wouldn't like it if someone did that to you.

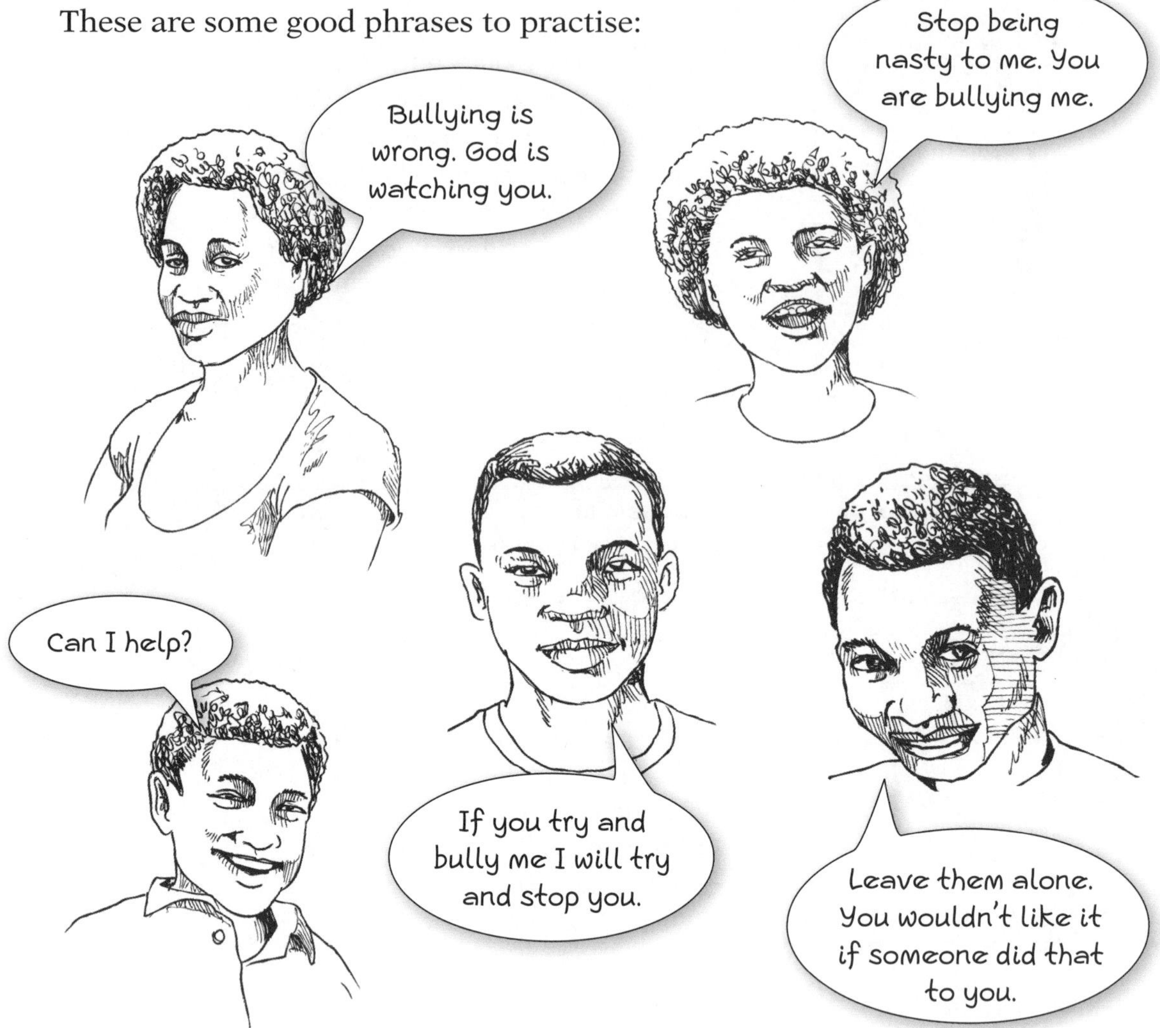

Romance in school

As you get older there is a good chance you will have a romantic relationship in school. Most schools have rules to keep you safe in these relationships.

Beware of having relationships with students who are much older or younger than you are.

See Chapter 9 for more information on safe romantic relationships.

Cults and generation names

Some schools have secret student groups. They are against the school rules. If you are a member of one of these groups you could be expelled.

Often the behaviour in these groups is bullying. You are forced to do something you would not normally do to be a part of the group. This is risky to your health, safety and education.

Here are some ways of dealing with cults:

- Say no confidently.
- Report the group to a counsellor or trusted teacher.
- Keep yourself busy with better activities like sport, music, drama and church.
- Help others to escape from the group.
- Be calm and sensible – a cult is just a form of peer pressure and bullying.
- Think of what your parents and younger brothers and sisters would say if they found out.

Activity 6.7 BULLYING PLAY SCRIPT

1 With your friends, write a play script about bullying and how it can be dealt with. Perform this for others.

2 Evaluate your play.
   - Is it realistic? Could it happen in your school?
   - Do the characters behave in a real-life way?
   - Are the solutions practical?

3 Discuss these questions with your class.
   - Why do some students bully others?
   - What can be the impact of bullying on young people?
   - What can we do to stop bullying?
   - How can we help the person being bullied?
   - How can we help the bully?
   - Is bullying a problem in your school?

4 Finally, list three personal actions you will take to improve your relationships with others in your school.

   For example, I pledge to speak to three younger students each break time and make sure they are all okay.

Chapter 7 Healthy relationships in your community

As you grow older, your roles and responsibilities in your community become more important. You will need to manage relationships with many different people in your community.

The same strategies for developing and maintaining relationships can be used with many of these people. For example:

- being respectful without blindly following other people's demands
- listening to other people's points of view and sharing your own
- being polite and constructive
- helping others
- treating other people how you would like to be treated
- staying calm and trying to solve problems without fighting
- asking for help when you need it
- sharing fairly.

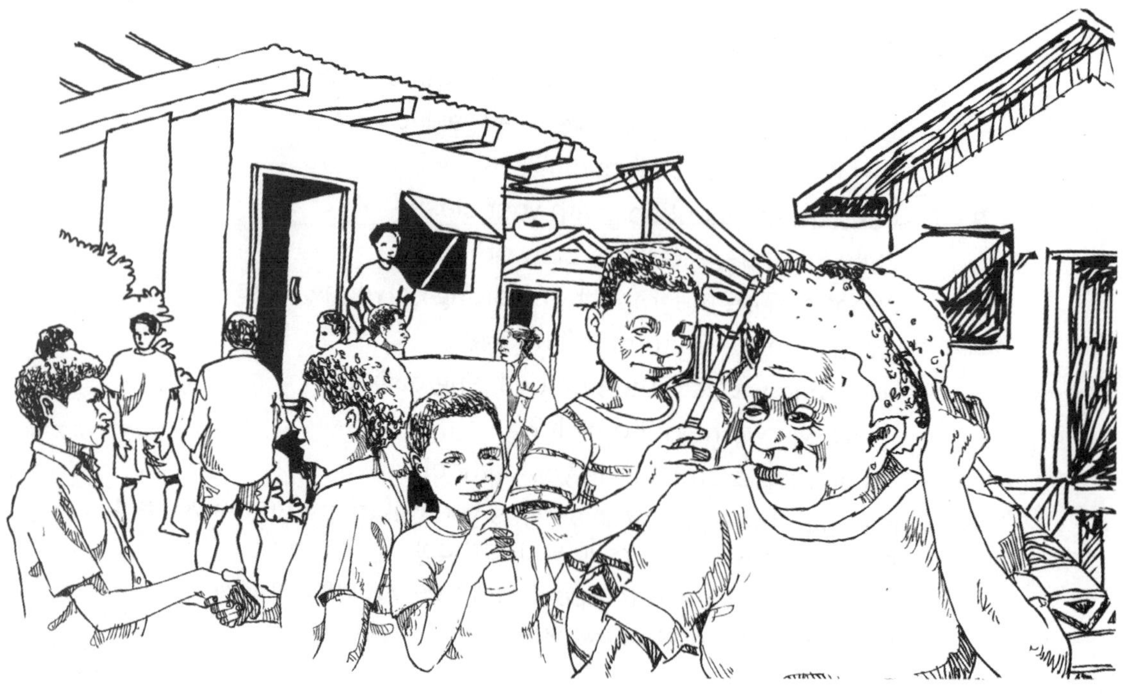

Relationships with your neighbours

Getting on with your neighbours is important whether you live in a traditional village, in a settlement or in an estate or compound.

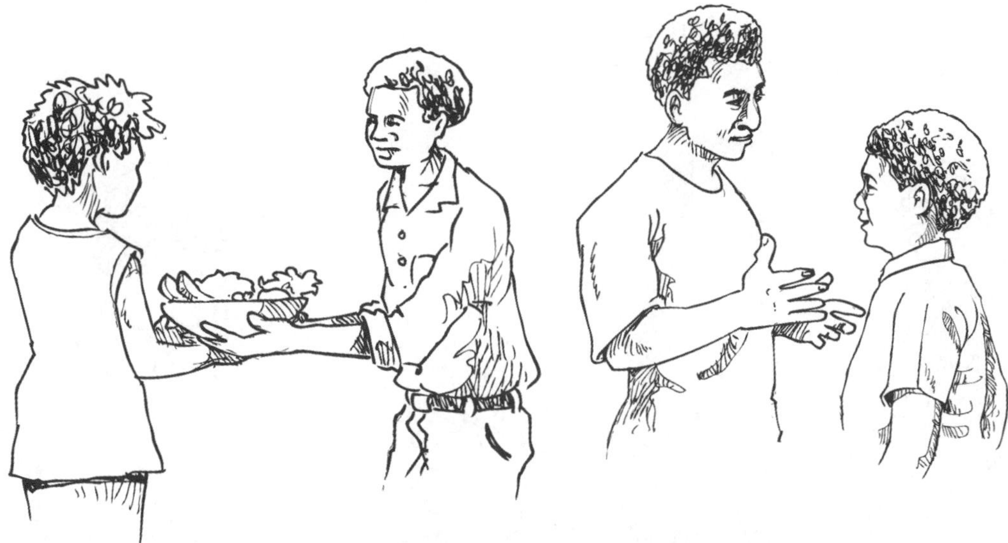

You can build good relationships with your neighbours by:

- being cheerful when you greet them
- taking time to talk and ask about their family
- helping them out when they need it
- sharing your food
- inviting them over
- not being noisy at night
- keeping control of your animals
- ensuring your garden is kept tidy.

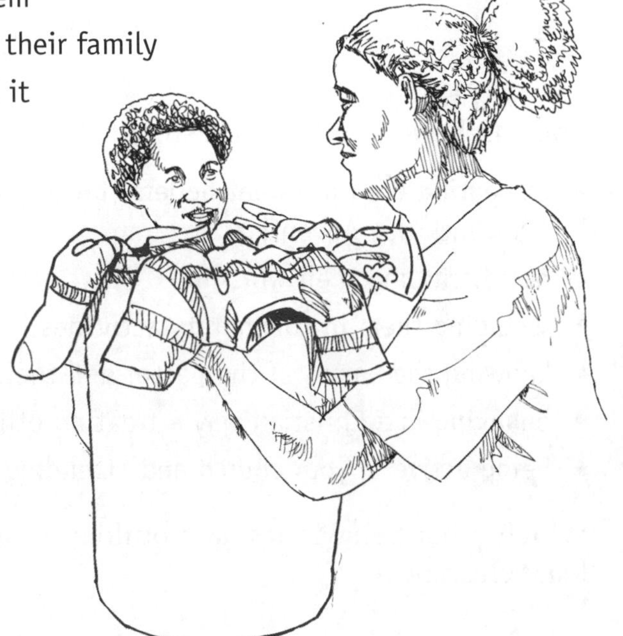

Which other behaviours help build strong relationships with your neighbours?

Relationships with your local churches

The church is an important part of community life. You might have several different churches in your community.

Whether you go to church regularly or not, it is important that you have a positive relationship with the church groups.

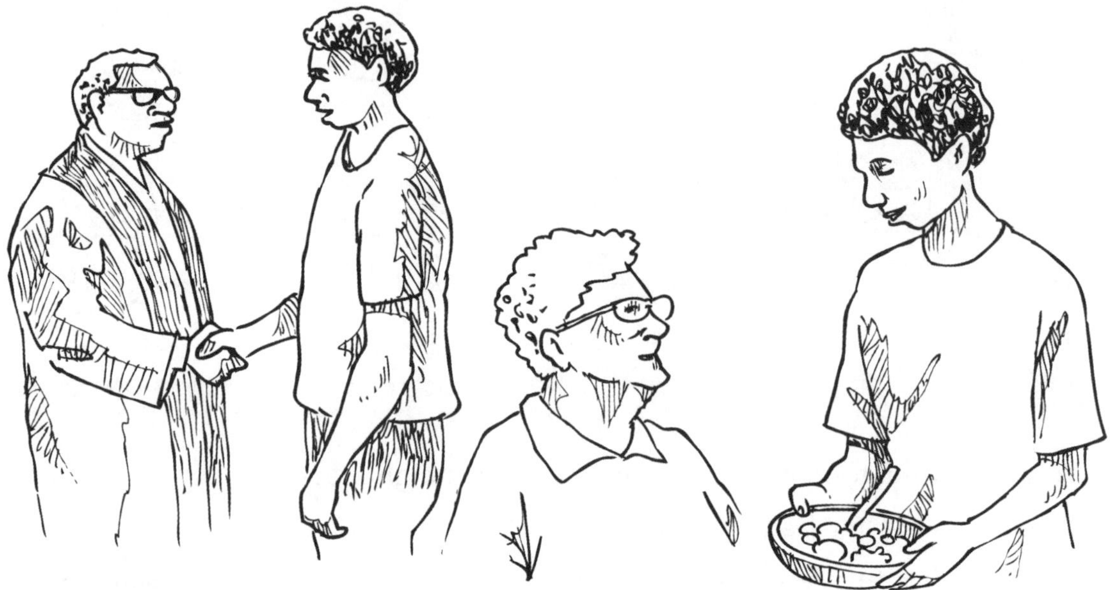

You can build good relationships with your local churches by:

- respecting their different beliefs (for example, not serving pork to a Seventh Day Adventist)
- not disturbing their worship
- including them in community activities
- knowing the names of the pastor and their family, and greeting them warmly
- behaving in a Christian way – treating others as you would like to be treated
- being active in your church and attending church regularly.

Which other behaviours help build strong relationships with your local churches?

Relationships with traditional and political leaders

Every community has councillors or traditional leaders. Sometimes these people are elected. In some cultures, there are also *bikmen* and *bikmeri* who have earned respect from the community.

As a young person, you have a right to contribute to the development of your community. You also have a responsibility to show respect to leaders and elders.

You can build good relationships with leaders by:

- listening to their views, being respectful and being polite in discussions
- making a positive contribution to development
- taking part in cultural traditions and exchanges
- voting wisely and independently
- refusing bribes and not expecting hand-outs
- speaking up for people who do not have a voice in the community
- working hard in school and the community.

Which other behaviours help build strong relationships with your leaders?

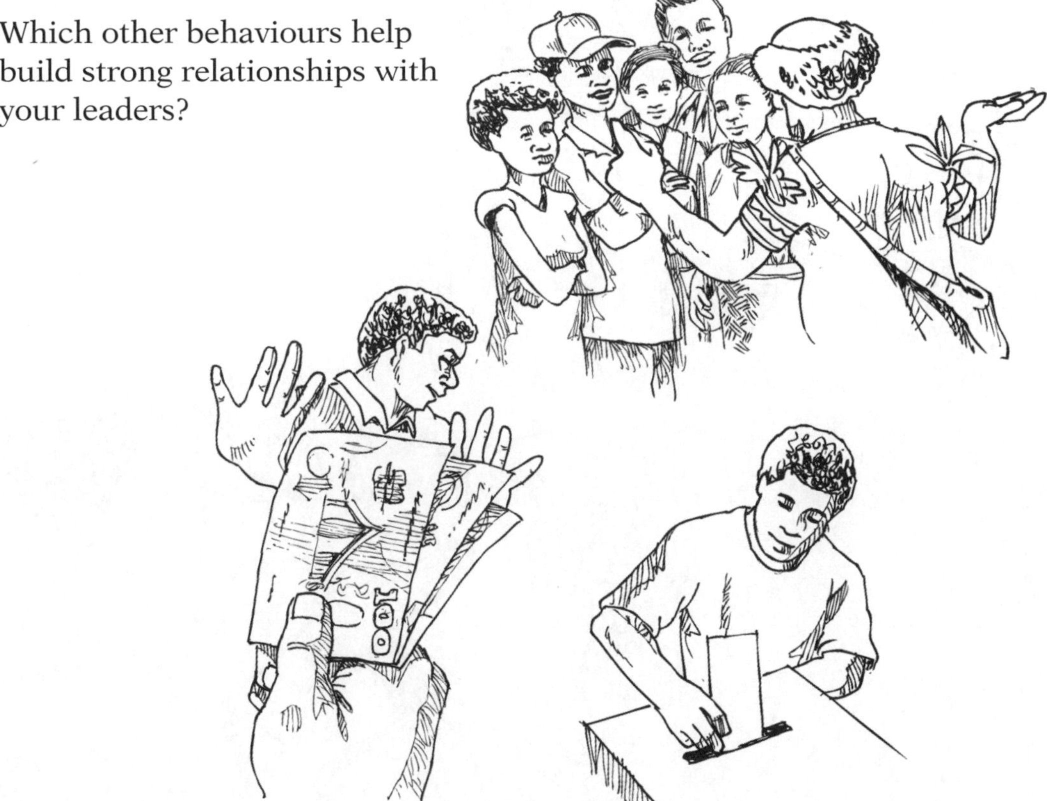

 Relationships with the police

You may have a local police officer. If they are based in your community, it is sensible to build a good relationship with them.

Sometimes police will visit your community after a crime has been committed. If they do visit, stay calm and be helpful. Make sure you get the name, rank and number of the officers.

You can build good relationships with the police by:

- getting to know your local police officer
- working hard to contribute to the development of your community
- stopping criminal behaviour in your community
- not getting drunk or using home-brew and marijuana
- ensuring your house is peaceful and free of abuse and violence
- reporting serious criminal activities.

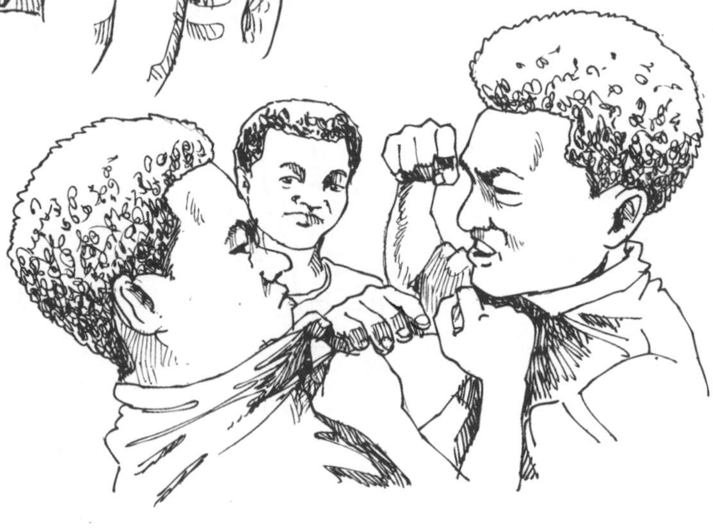

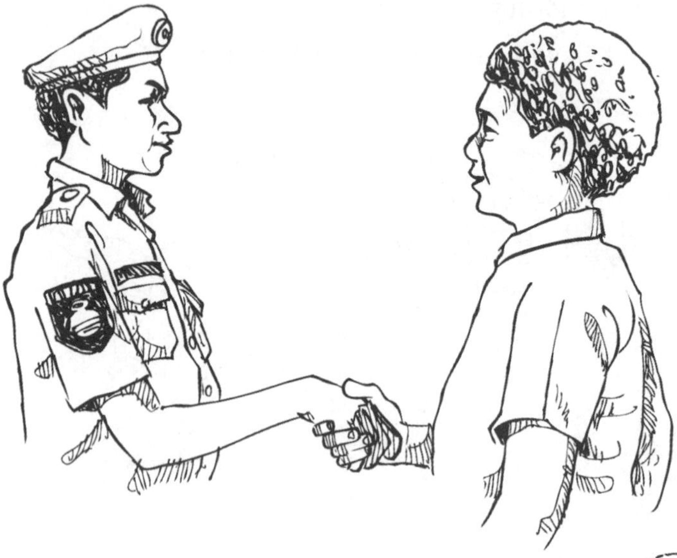

 Relationships with your work colleagues

Going to work is an important responsibility. If you work hard and behave well at work, you will get a good reference for any future job and you are more likely to be promoted.

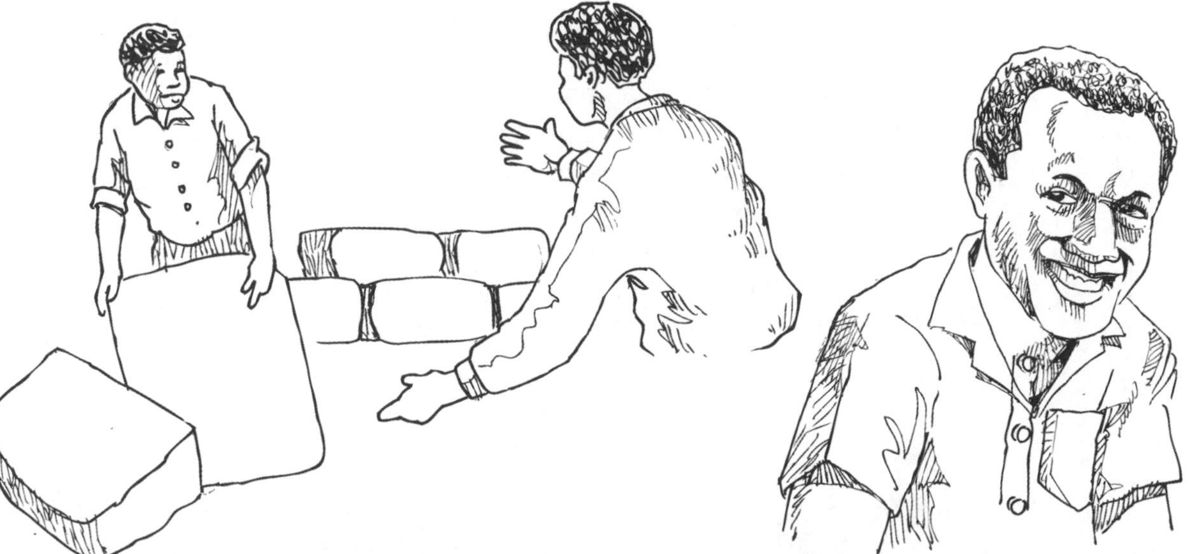

You can build good relationships with your work colleagues by:

- being punctual
- working hard, doing your job well and taking the initiative
- following instructions sensibly
- getting to know your workmates
- being honest and trustworthy
- being neat and sober and not chewing or smoking
- understanding the business you are working for.

Which other behaviours help build strong relationships with your work colleagues and employer?

Activity 7.1 OTHER IMPORTANT RELATIONSHIPS IN YOUR COMMUNITY

1 List at least two other important groups in the community with which you will need to build a healthy relationship. For example, PMV crews, health workers, trade store owner, expatriates, the coach of a sports team.

2 For each group, complete a page like the previous ones with an illustration and a list of behaviours which would help improve your relationship with that group.

3 Which other groups can young people join? Why are these groups important in helping young people develop? For example, scouts, girl guides, church youth groups, sports teams.

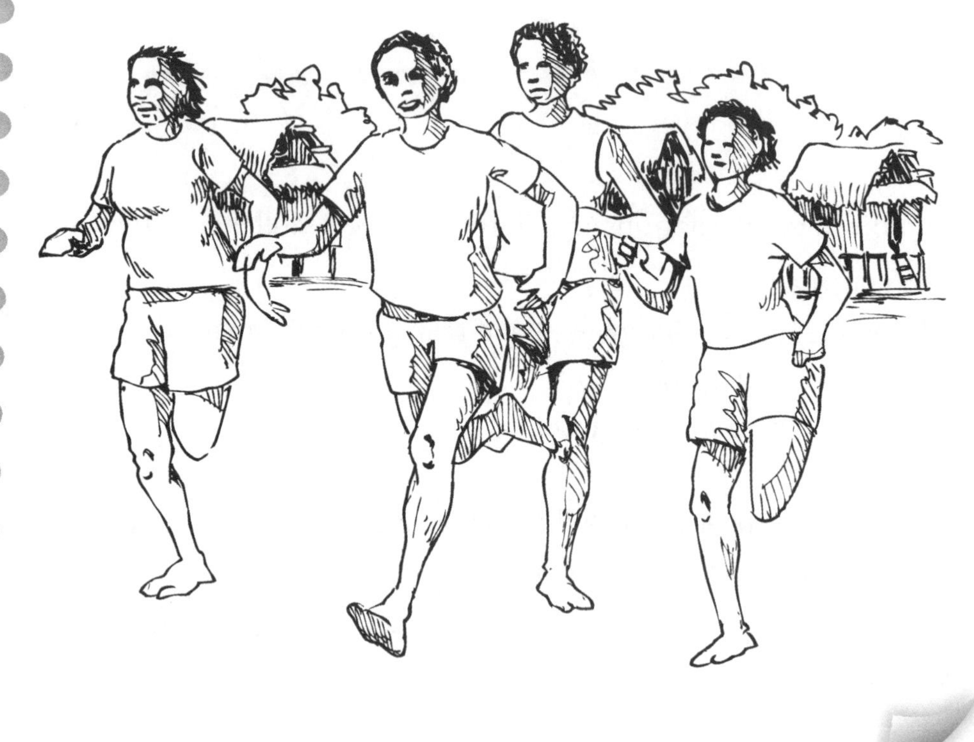

Changing roles and responsibilities

You can become a leader in your community in many ways. Being a role model for younger people, getting a good education, speaking up against injustice and helping others are all parts of being a responsible adult.

Showing you can build strong relationships is a step towards earning more respect and responsibility in your community.

Activity 7.2 YOUR ROLE IN YOUR COMMUNITY

Complete these personal goals:

1 I will help people in my community by ...
2 I will earn the respect of my community by ...
3 I will prevent conflicts in my community by ...
4 I will be a good neighbour by ...
5 I will be a good role model by ...
6 My own role models will be ...
7 When people in my community describe me, I want them to say I am ...

Chapter 8 Keeping safe

As you grow older, you will develop and experience many different kinds of relationships. It is important to understand what is **acceptable behaviour** and what is **unacceptable behaviour** in each of these relationships. It is also important to learn skills that will help you avoid relationships that might put you at risk.

The diagram on the next page will help you to identify different kinds of relationships. Each bigger circle represents a different kind of relationship.

Circle 1 The person at the centre of the circle is you. If someone else is in the circle with you, it is someone you are sharing your body with – someone you are sexually active with. That person must be invited into your circle.

Circle 2 This circle includes people who you love, trust and share your life with. This might include immediate family members, partners and best friends.

Circle 3 This circle includes people who you know well, but not as well as those in circle 2. This circle might include close friends and relatives.

Circle 4 This circle includes people who you regularly come into contact with. You do not share an emotional relationship with them, but you do spend time with them on a regular basis. This might include teachers, doctors, school mates and team mates.

Circle 5 This circle includes people who you come into contact with only once in a while. You do not have an emotional or social relationship with them. You treat them politely and with respect. This might include PMV drivers, service providers and shop workers.

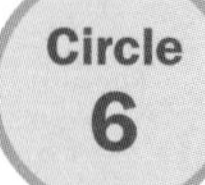

This circle includes everybody else.

The 'out' circle includes people who you have strong disagreements with or dislike for. This may be a permanent situation or a temporary situation. This might include an ex-partner or person with whom you have had a serious argument, or a person who has betrayed your trust.

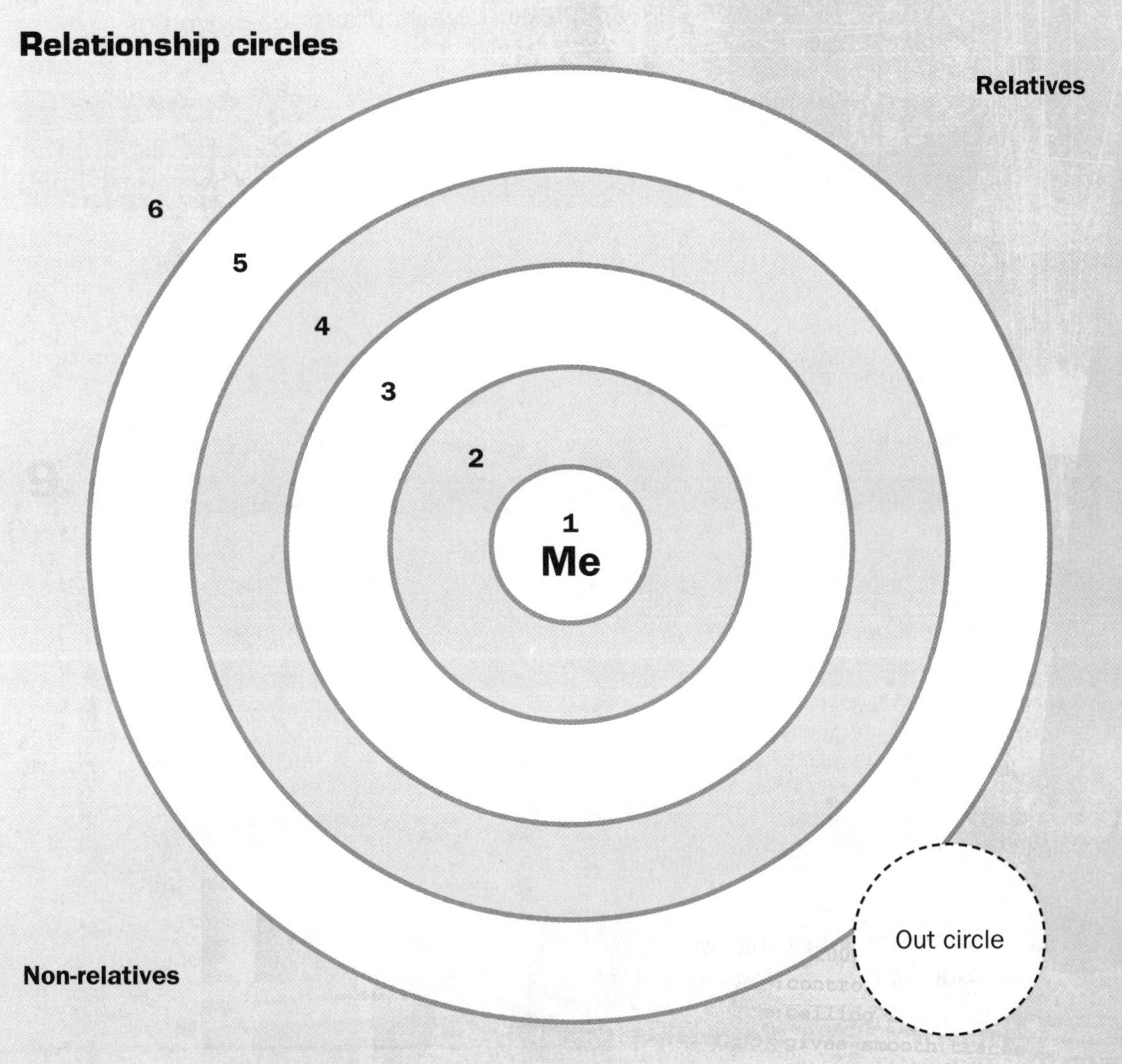

It is possible for people to move from one circle to another. For example, your best friend may have started out as a stranger (circle 6), but as you got to know them and developed trust and respect for them, they moved into a closer circle.

Activity 8.1 ACCEPTABLE AND UNACCEPTABLE BEHAVIOUR

Look at the relationship circles on the previous page. Identify people from your own life who fit into each of these circles. List some acceptable and unacceptable behaviours for each kind of relationship.

	Person	Acceptable behaviour	Unacceptable behaviour
1	• me • partner	• •	• •
2	• partner • parents	• hug •	• •
3	• uncle •	• •	• sexual touching •
4	• teachers •	• •	• hitting •
5	• PMV drivers •	• handshake •	• sexual touching •

Compare your table with your friends' tables.

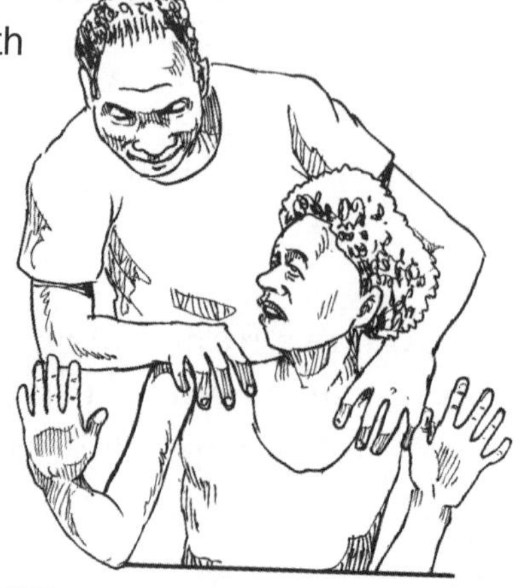

Sexual abuse

Each of your relationships is put into a particular circle based on the trust, respect and affection you have for that person. It is your choice who you put in which circle and when you choose to put them there.

It is your right to decide who you are sexually active with. You always have the right to refuse sexual contact of any kind and to say no or stop at any time. You are the only person who has the right to decide who will be in your 'me' circle.

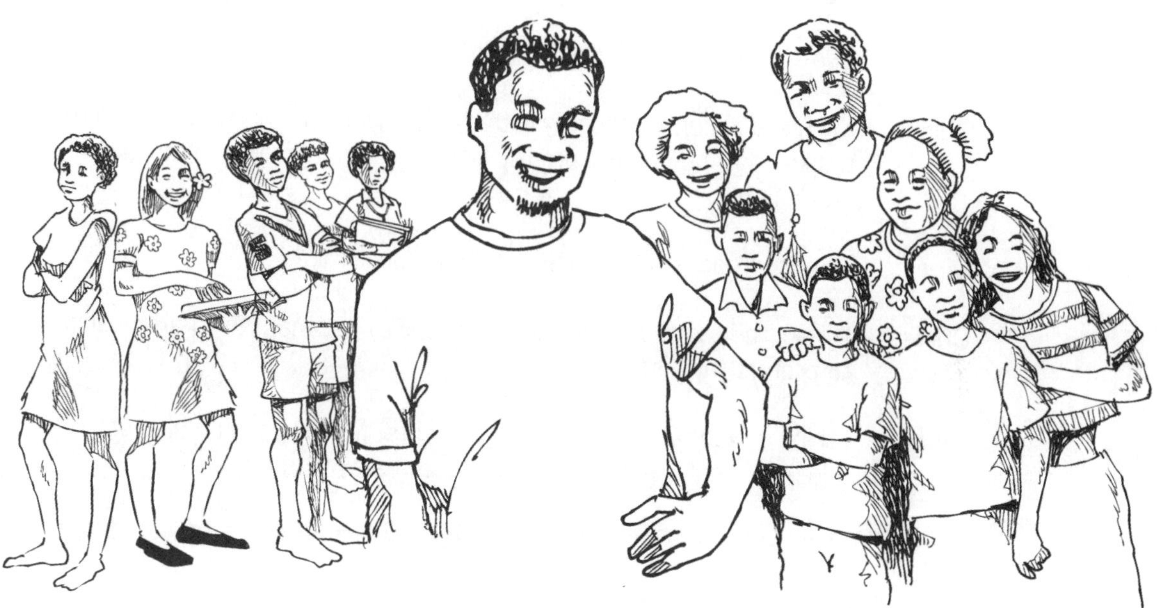

There are certain people who should never be sexually active with you. They should never be in your 'me' circle. Nobody from the relatives side of your relationship circle should be in your 'me' circle. Sexual activity of any kind should only be with someone from the non-relatives side. If a relative touches you in a sexual manner this is **sexual abuse**.

If a person forces themselves into your 'me' circle this is also sexual abuse. If a person forces you to have sex with them this is **rape**. Often, a person who tries to do this comes from circle 2 or 3 and could be a friend or relative.

People in positions of authority, such as teachers, doctors and police, should never be sexually active with you or in your 'me' circle. This is an abuse of their power.

Activity 8.2 CASE STUDIES

1 Read the different scenarios below. For each situation identify the unacceptable behaviour and the strategy used to remove the danger.

Case study 1: In the family

Mary: Chris, what's wrong? You look worried.

Chris: My uncle is coming to stay with the family for the holidays. When he drinks a lot, he sneaks into my sister's room. He tries to touch her and kiss her.

Mary: This is wrong. Do your parents know about this?

Chris: I'm scared to tell my parents in case they get mad. But I also want to protect my sister.

Mary: I think it is time you talk to your parents. Maybe you can also get a lock for your sister's door, or she can stay with a friend.

Chris: Thanks, Mary. Those are good ideas. I will try them.

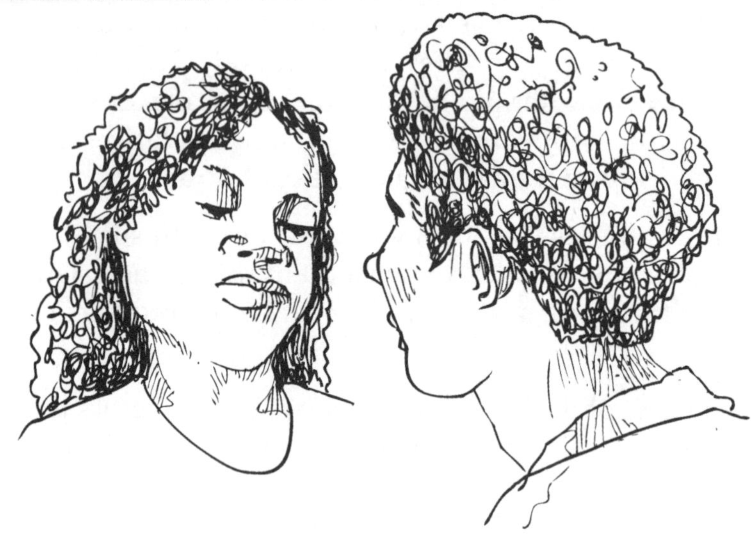

Case study 2: In school

George: Anne, a bunch of us are playing volleyball after school. Do you want to come?

Anne: Thanks, but I am going to talk to Mr Smith about my maths test. He said I could talk to him about improving my grades.

George: Be careful, Anne. I know another girl who Mr Smith helped. He told the girl that if she touched him and kissed him, he would raise her grades.

Anne: Oh, no. Now I'm scared. But I really need to pass maths.

George: I can come with you, if you like, or maybe you can ask another teacher to go with you.

Anne: That's a good idea, George. I will ask Ms Mita to go with me.

2 What would you do if you or someone you knew were in Anne or Mary's situation?

3 Is there an adult in your family or community you could go to for assistance and support if you find yourself in this situation?

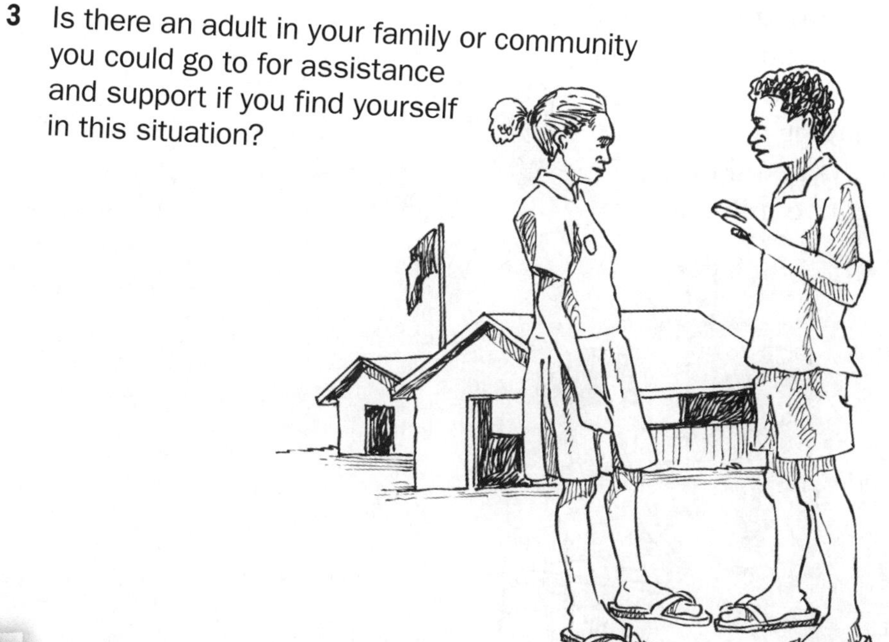

Peer pressure

During puberty and adolescence, having a group of friends of similar age is important. Young people can support one another through the many changes they experience during this time. They can encourage one another to try new things and protect one another from abuse or peer pressure.

Peer pressure can be good and bad. Peer pressure is how someone is influenced by other people's behaviour. When you are growing up, different people will influence the decisions you make in different ways.

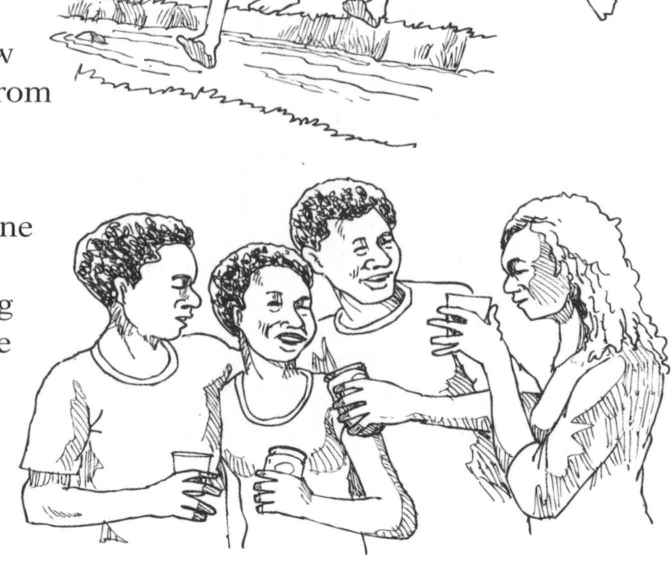

Most young people feel it is important for them to belong to a group of friends and to 'fit in'. Friends can influence your behaviour in both good and bad ways. It is important for young people to recognise when their friends are having a positive influence and when they are having a negative influence.

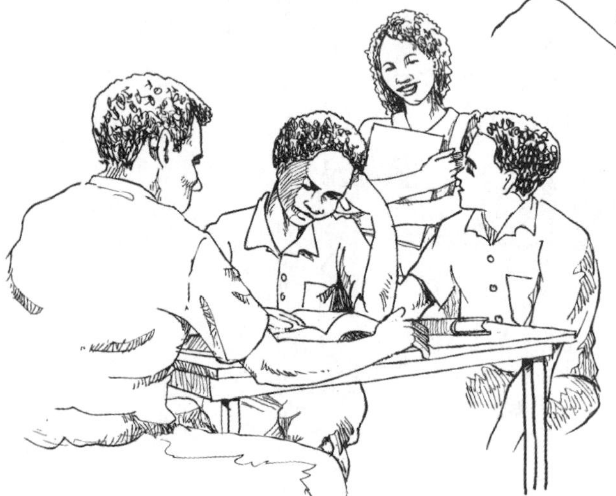

Activity 8.3 THE GOOD AND BAD IMPACTS OF PEER PRESSURE

Think of times when your friends influenced decisions you made. Was their influence good or bad? What was the result of your decision?

For example:

Decision	Good or bad influence?	Impact
Including a new person in our group of friends	Good	I met someone new and made a new friend.
Staying late in town	Bad	My parents were angry. I didn't finish my homework.

At one point or another, most young people will experience peer pressure. There are many things that young people can do to prepare themselves for harmful peer pressure. The best way to avoid peer pressure is to choose friends with similar values to you and who respect your opinions and decisions.

It is also important to be comfortable with who you are and what you are comfortable with. Consider your answers to Activities 1.1, 2.3, 3.3 and 5.1. Your answers reflect your values and what is important to you.

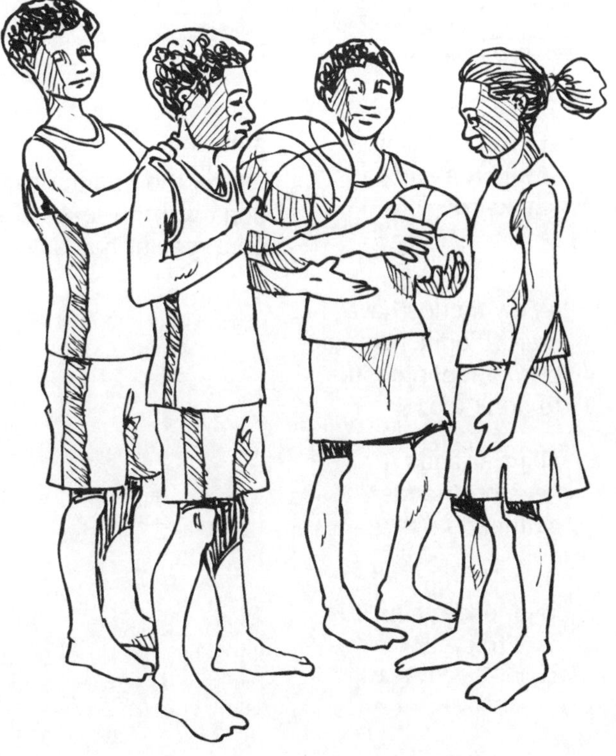

Activity 8.4 PLANNING FOR PEER PRESSURE

The following are common situations where young people experience harmful peer pressure. Consider each situation. What would you be comfortable doing and not doing in each situation? What strategies could you use to avoid or get out of this situation?

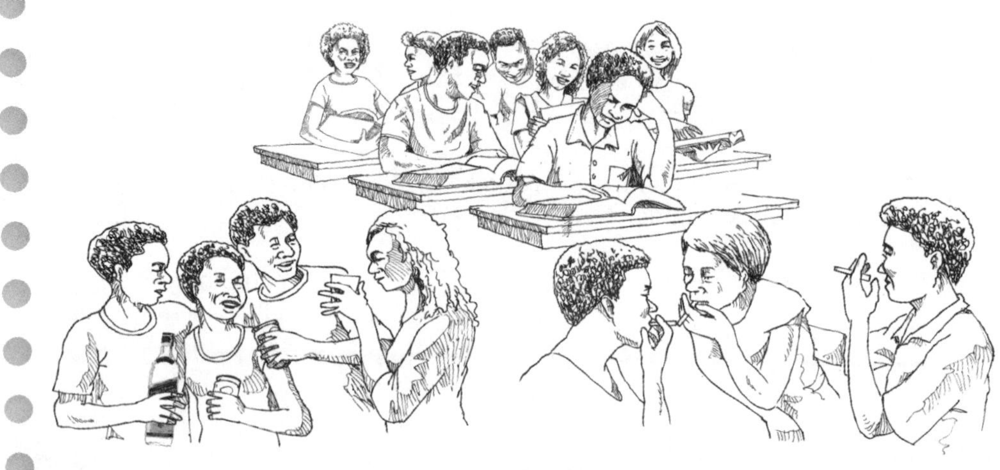

Situation	Knowing your limits	Coping strategies
All my friends have started smoking. I feel pressure to smoke too.	I am curious and might try smoking. I know the health risks and don't want to take up smoking on a regular basis.	Say: 'No thanks, I tried it, but I don't think it's for me.' Say: 'No thanks, I don't want to have yellow teeth and bad breath.'
All my friends have started drinking home brew. I feel pressure to drink too.		
All my friends have boyfriends/ girlfriends.		
My friends think it is cool to steal.		

Role models

A role model is someone whose behaviour and relationships with others sets an example for other people to follow. Role models often have many of the positive and healthy values and behaviours that we have discussed in earlier chapters. They have healthy relationships with their families, communities and colleagues that are based on respect, trust and understanding.

Identifying a role model for healthy relationships is a good way for young people to learn what healthy and safe relationships are. Young people can learn by example from role models by watching how they treat others, listening to how they communicate with others, and observing how they handle disagreements. Young people can also speak to role models about challenges they might be experiencing in their relationships and get advice and support to handle these challenges.

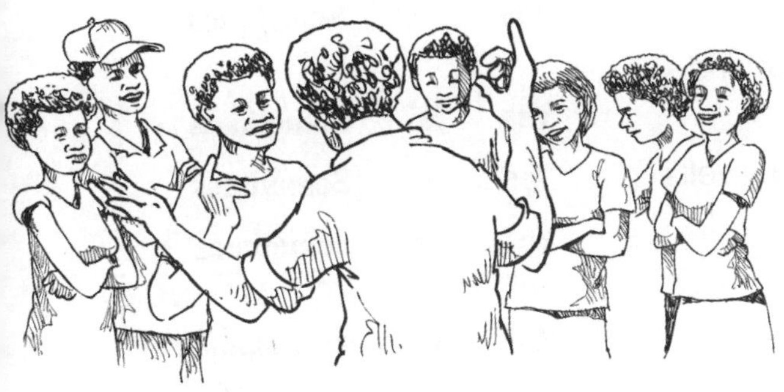

A role model is often older than the person they provide advice to. Here are some examples of role models:

- a senior student can be a role model to a younger student
- an older sibling can be a role model to a younger sibling
- a teacher can be a role model to a class of students
- an athlete can be a role model
- a community leader or parent can be a role model.

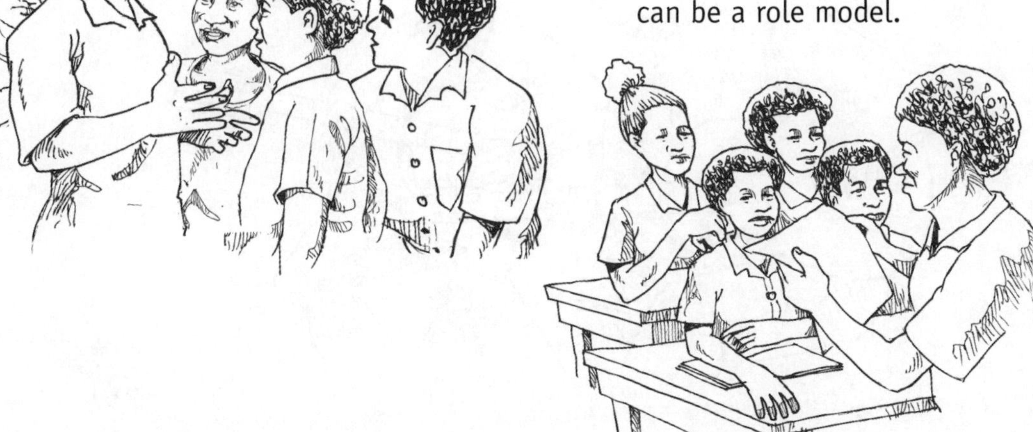

Activity 8.5 ARE YOU A GOOD ROLE MODEL?

You can be a role model too! Often people are role models without even knowing it. If you are an older sibling or senior student, then the chances are that someone is watching how you behave and treat others.

Are you a good role model? Consider the following questions.

1	Do you value others?	**Yes**	**No**	**Sometimes**
2	Do you treat people with respect?	**Yes**	**No**	**Sometimes**
3	Do you pressure friends to do things?	**Yes**	**No**	**Sometimes**
4	Do you help friends and family with homework or housework?	**Yes**	**No**	**Sometimes**
5	Do you get angry easily?	**Yes**	**No**	**Sometimes**
6	Do you argue a lot?	**Yes**	**No**	**Sometimes**
7	Do you talk about people behind their back?	**Yes**	**No**	**Sometimes**
8	Do you support friends to do well?	**Yes**	**No**	**Sometimes**
9	Do you keep your promises?	**Yes**	**No**	**Sometimes**
10	Do you admit your mistakes and apologise?	**Yes**	**No**	**Sometimes**

How can you change your behaviour so that you become a good role model?

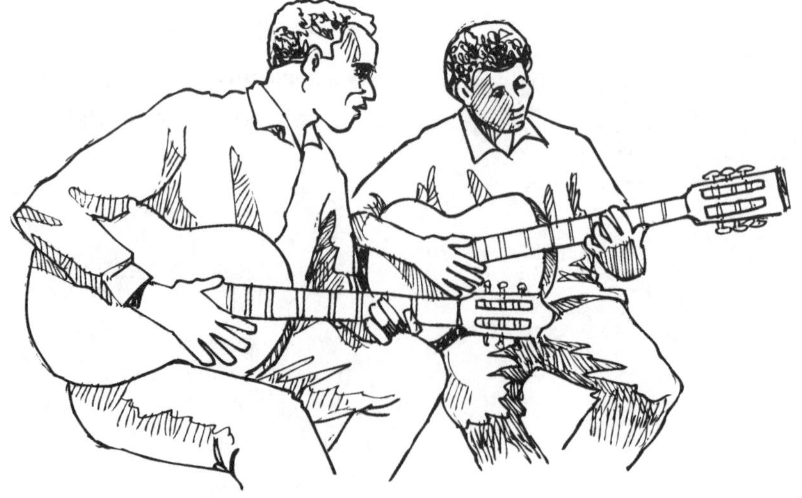

Peer educators

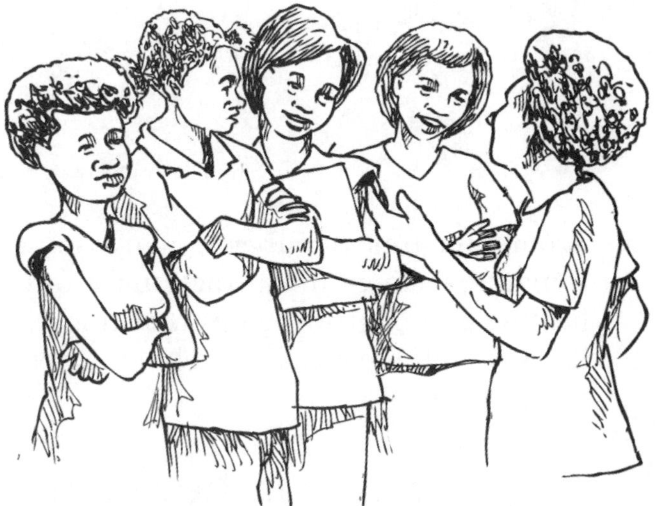

Often young people find it easier to talk to their peers. A **peer educator** is someone who is the same age and sex as you, or has similar interests. They usually receive some training to learn how to share information with their peers.

Many schools have peer education programs. Some students are selected to receive additional training. They are usually confident, mature and trustworthy. Once they have been trained, they are asked to discuss different topics with their peers, or conduct different activities. Peer educators can be a great source of information about relationships, safe behaviours and other issues that young people face.

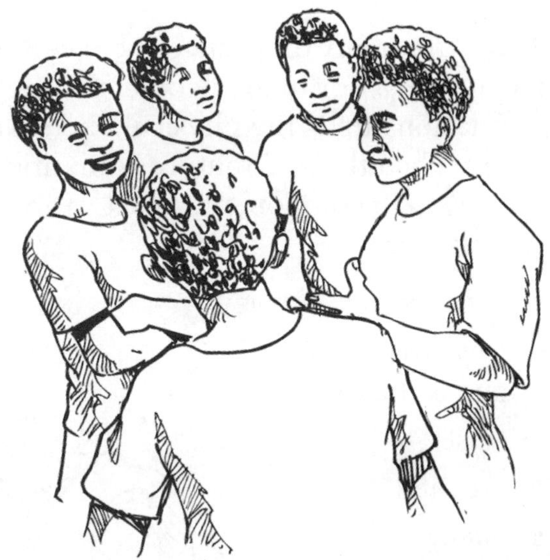

Chapter 9 Safe romantic relationships

Around the time of puberty, many young people start to experience romantic feelings and attraction for other people. This is a natural and healthy part of growing up. Learning the skills to develop and maintain healthy and safe romantic relationships will help you to live a happy and healthy life.

Differences between romantic relationships and friendships

There are many differences between romantic relationships and friendships. For many people, the biggest difference in these two types of relationship is the physical and sexual aspect of the relationship. If you are in a healthy and mature romantic relationship, the sexual aspect is only a small component. Apart from sexual activity, romantic relationships can also bring:

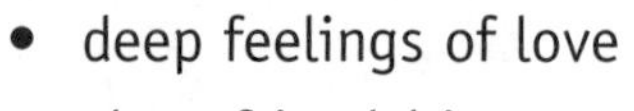

- deep feelings of love
- close friendship and partnership
- trust
- security
- family
- comfort
- understanding
- support.

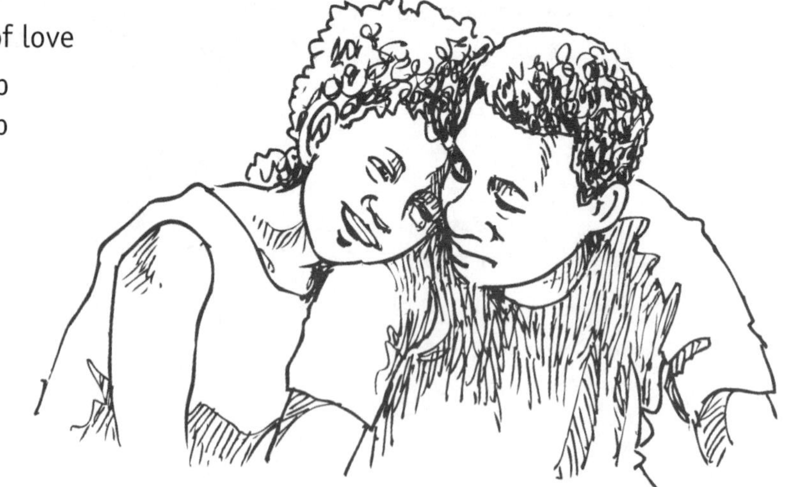

Each person has a different idea of what a romantic relationship is. Before you get involved in a romantic relationship, it is important for you to know what you want and expect from a romantic relationship and from your romantic partner. This will help you to choose a suitable partner and to make healthy decisions about your relationship.

Activity 9.1 WHAT ARE YOU LOOKING FOR?

1 What do different people look for in a partner? Read these statements with a group of peers. Do you agree with their reasons?

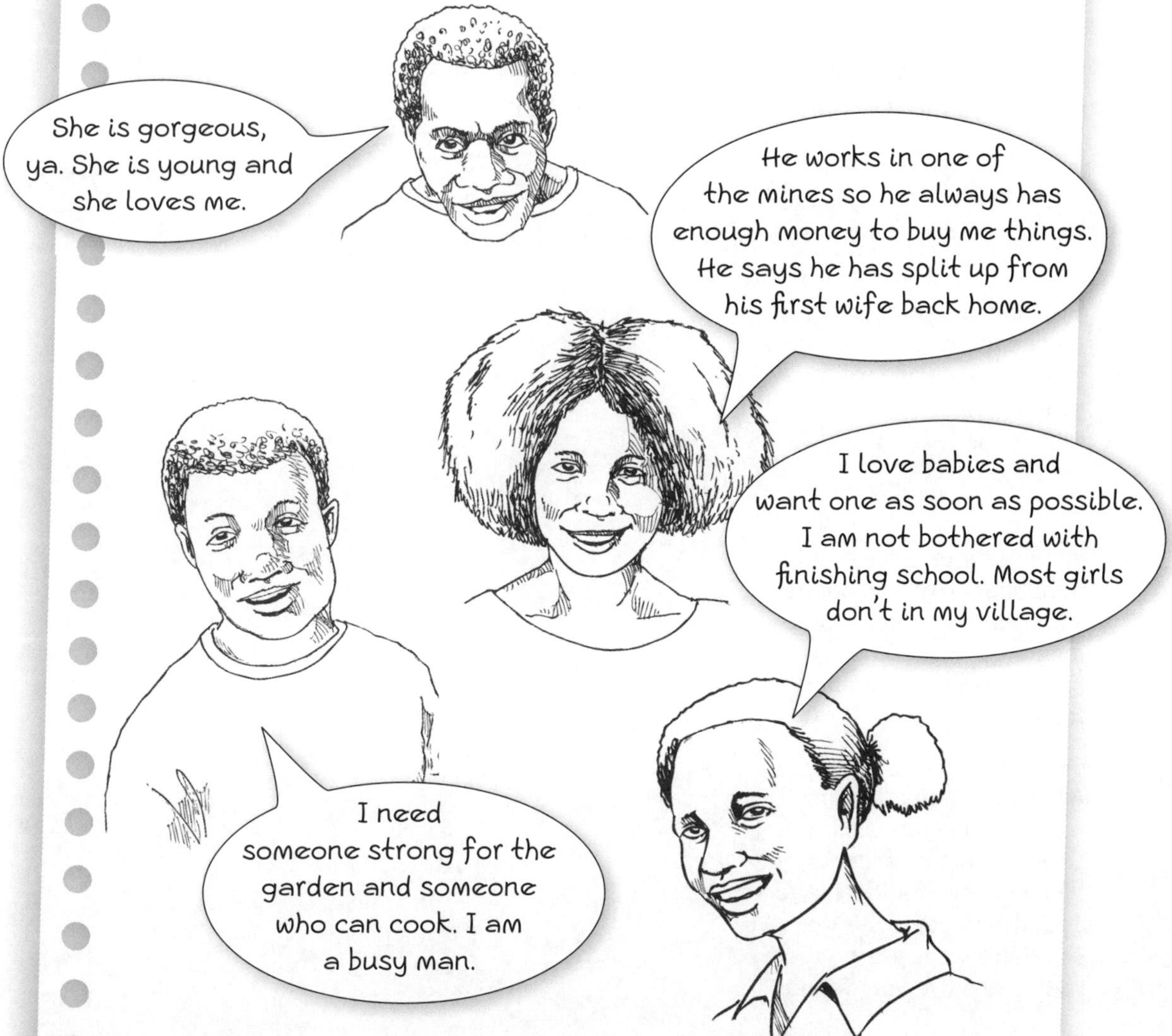

2 List what you and your friends look for in a partner. Which are the most important features?

3 Now compare your list with a group of students of the opposite sex. What do you notice about what they look for in a husband or wife or boyfriend or girlfriend?

Deciding to get involved in a romantic relationship is an important decision. It is something that you should think about and consider carefully.

Activity 9.2 CHOICES AND CONSEQUENCES

Consider the following situations and choices. Think about the possible consequences of each choice and what might happen as a result. Complete this table with a friend.

Choice	Consequences	Result
You decide to go out with someone because they have lots of money and will give you presents.		
You decide to start a relationship with someone you have known for a very long time, who you trust and have developed romantic feelings for.		
All of your friends are in romantic relationships and think you are strange for not being in one. You decide to go out with someone that you don't really like so that you can be like your friends.		
There isn't really anyone who you want to have a romantic relationship with, but you want to learn more about sex. You decide to go out with someone who likes you, but who you don't really like.		

For many people, a sexual relationship is a big part of a romantic relationship, but being in a romantic relationship does not mean that you have to have sex. Deciding when to have sex or what kind of sexual activities you want to do is something only you can decide. It is important to discuss with your partner what sexual activities you are comfortable with and what sexual activities you are not comfortable with. As you become closer with your partner your comfort level may change, but only you can decide that.

Activity 9.3 YES, NO, MAYBE

It is important to know your own sexual boundaries before getting involved in a romantic relationship. This will help you to tell your partner.

Consider the following physical and sexual activities. Which ones are you comfortable with (Yes)? Which ones are you not comfortable with (No)? And which ones aren't you sure about (Maybe)?

Physical or sexual activity	Yes, no, maybe
Having a partner touch me lovingly without asking first	
Holding hands with a partner in public	
Kissing in public	
Having my shirt/top off with a partner	
Having my pants/bottoms off with a partner	
Being naked with a partner	
Kissing with closed mouth	
Kissing with open mouth	
Having a partner touch my chest, breasts or nipples	
Touching a partner's chest, breasts or nipples	
Having a partner touch my penis or vulva	
Touching a partner's penis or vulva	
Having sexual intercourse with a partner	
Discussing sexual history with a partner	
Discussing condom use with a partner	

As a young person, you will start to make your own decisions about your romantic, physical and sexual relationships. Learning how to communicate with your partner about your goals, expectations and boundaries is an important skill to have.

Activity 9.4 ROLE PLAY

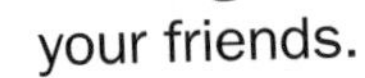

With a group of friends, consider the following situations. Write a dialogue to resolve the situation. Act out these situations with your friends.

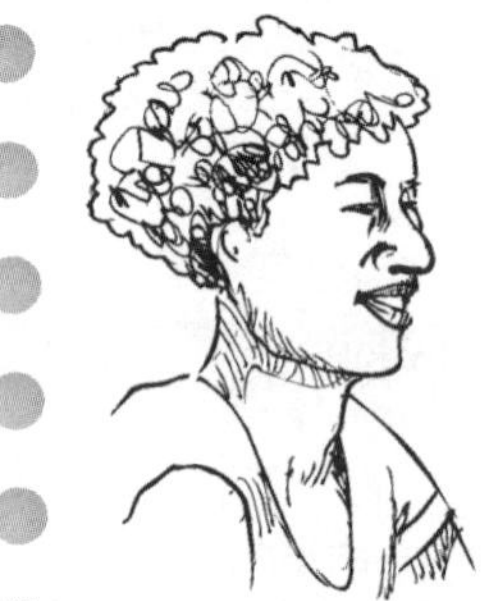

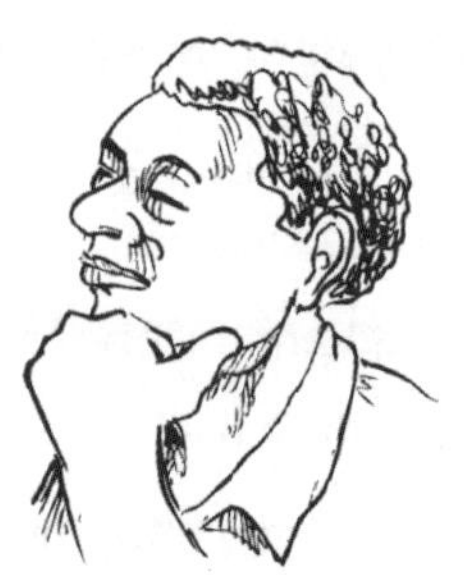

Scene 1

Fidelis and Susan have been going out for a long time. They love and trust one another and feel that they are ready to have sex for the first time. Susan knows that Fidelis has had other partners and is concerned about STIs. She is also concerned about getting pregnant.

Scene 2

Alex and Serah have been going out for a long time. After high school Alex will go to Lae for university and Serah will go to Port Moresby for university. Serah is an active member in her church, and wants to wait until she gets married to have sex. Alex wants to have sex soon. Both agree that they are too young to get married.

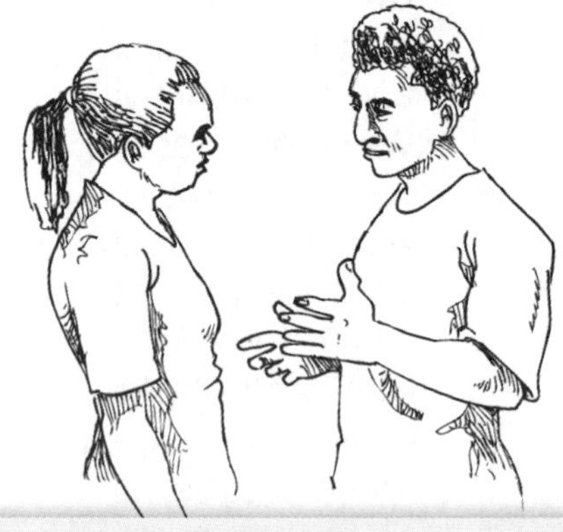

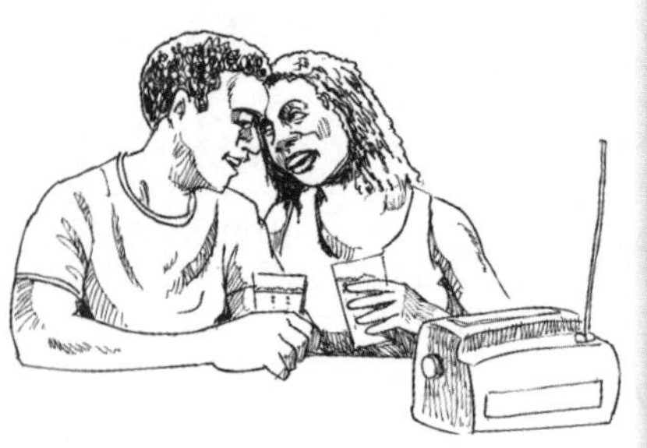

Scene 3

Julius and Daisy have only known each other for a short time. They are very attracted to each other. They like to hang out together and drink beers and listen to music. Usually they end by fooling around. The last time, they came very close to having sex, but Julius's friend called. Julius likes Daisy and the sexual activity. Daisy is concerned that things are moving too fast. They have plans to see each other again tonight.

Unhealthy romantic relationships

Healthy relationships should be based on love, respect and trust. Each person in the relationship should have the freedom to make their own choices and set their own boundaries.

Unhealthy romantic relationships happen when one person in the relationship has more control or power over the other person in the relationship. The person who is not in control may feel pressured to act in a certain way, or to do sexual activities that they are not comfortable with. This is abuse. This abuse can be emotional, mental or physical.

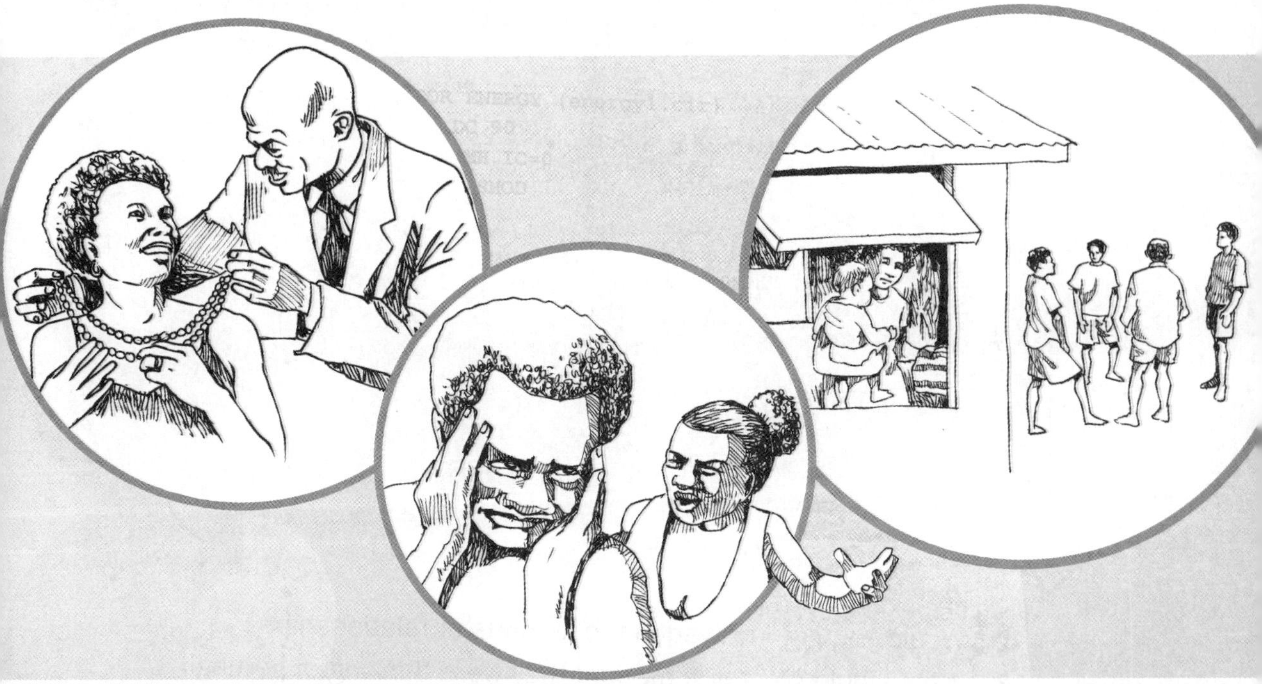

Effects of alcohol

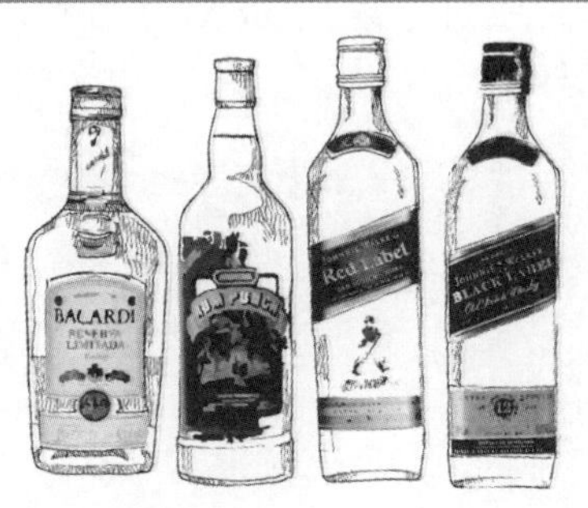

When people drink alcohol they can become loud and aggressive. They may behave differently and make choices that they wouldn't otherwise make. Drinking large amounts of alcohol can often lead to unsafe situations and behaviours. Drinking alcohol is not an excuse for poor behaviour.

If you drink, do so responsibly. If you think that you might be in an unsafe situation because of your partner's drinking, find a safe place to stay until your partner is sober.

Activity 9.5 WHAT DO YOU THINK?

Sugar daddies and relationships between older people and younger people are common in PNG.

1 Work with your friends to fill in the table below.

Type of relationship	Why do people get involved in this kind of relationship?	What is most likely to happen to the person with less control in this relationship?
Sugar daddies	• • •	• • •
Older man/woman going out with much younger person	• • •	• • •

2 Would you get involved in these kinds of relationships?

3 What would you tell a friend if they were thinking of getting involved in this kind of relationship?

Getting out of an unhealthy relationship can be very difficult. Staying in an unhealthy relationship can be unsafe and dangerous for you, your children and other family members.

Activity 9.6 SAFETY PLAN

Work with your friends to develop a safety plan to use if you find yourself in an unhealthy relationship.

- Who can you tell?
- Where can you go?
- What actions can you take?

How can you support friends or family members who are in unhealthy relationships?

Conflict resolution in romantic relationships

Even the happiest couples in the healthiest of relationships will have disagreements from time to time. This is normal. How a couple handles their disagreements is very important.

Some strategies for handing conflicts include:

- acknowledging and identifying the source of conflict in a timely manner
- giving your partner opportunities to express their feelings openly and honestly
- listening to your partner attentively
- expressing hurt or anger about a behaviour, not the person
- acting with maturity, respect and understanding
- accepting responsibility for poor behaviour
- solving problems and agreeing to solutions together
- valuing your partner's opinion.

Chapter 10 Healthy marriage

There are many different types of marriages in PNG cultures. Some are arranged marriages and some are marriages based on mutual attraction and independent choice. Other marriages are formally recognised in a church or by the law and some are informal long-term relationships. These relationships can be arranged in different ways depending on culture, religious beliefs or what has happened in a person's life.

 Type of marriage

Traditional marriage

Usually with a traditional ceremony such as bride price or shell exchange.

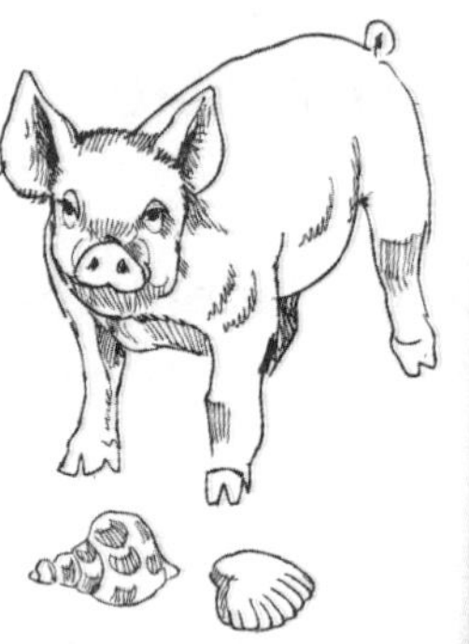

Church marriage

When a couple are married in church.

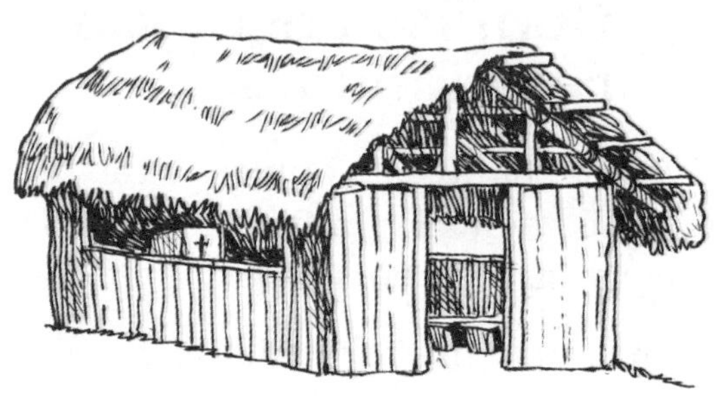

Civil marriage

When a couple are legally married but there is no religious or cultural ceremony.

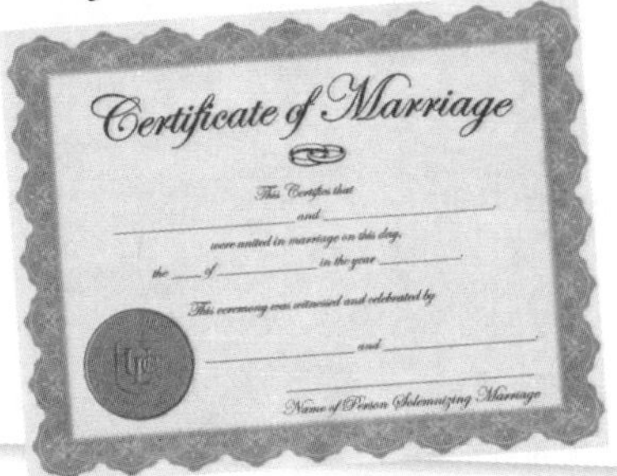

Certificate of Marriage

This Certifies that
and
were united in marriage on this day,
the ___ of ___ in the year ___
This ceremony was witnessed and celebrated by
and
Name of Person Solemnizing Marriage

De facto marriage

When a couple live together and have a long-term relationship (perhaps with children) but never marry.

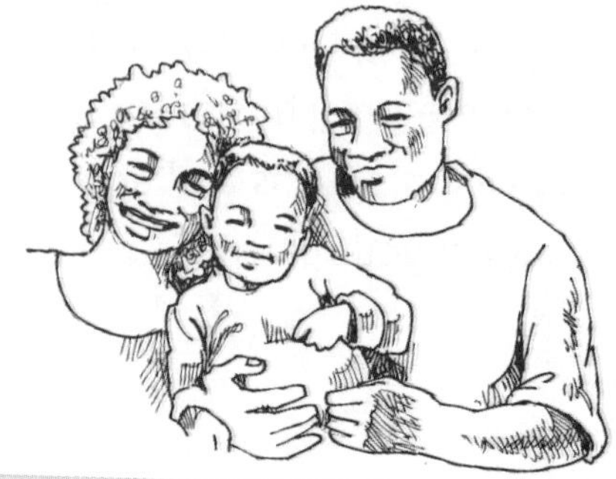

Reason for marriage

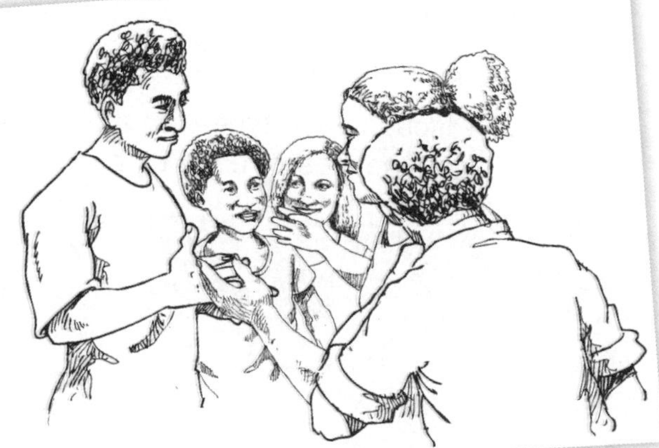

Arranged marriage

This is a traditional type of marriage where the families decide who marries.

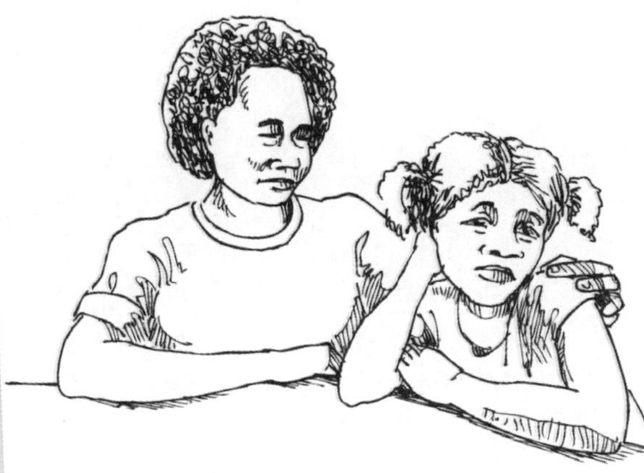

Marriage of convenience or marriage of survival

This is a relationship where one member of the couple needs the other to survive. Sometimes other kinds of marriage are really marriages of survival.

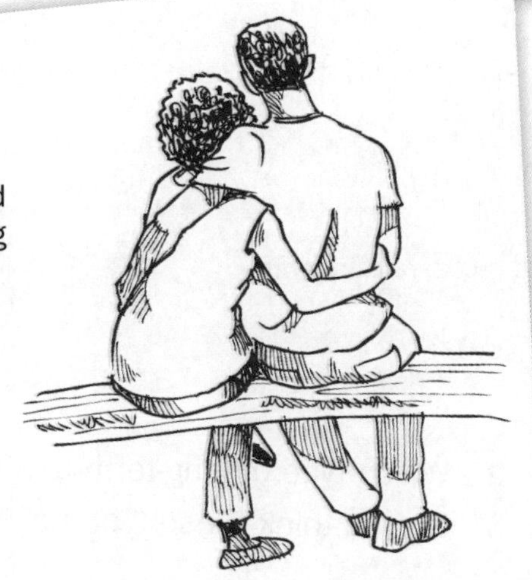

Love marriage

This is a type of marriage where the man and woman decide to marry based on deep loving feelings that they have for one another. They have similar life goals, interests and values.

Activity 10.1 DIFFERENT TYPES OF RELATIONSHIPS AND MARRIAGES

There are many different types of marriages or long-term relationships.

1 Discuss each type with a friend. What are the strengths and weaknesses of each type of marriage/long-term relationship?

Type of marriage/ relationship	Strengths	Weaknesses
Traditional marriage		
Love marriage		
De facto marriage		
Arranged marriage		
Marriage of survival		
Polygamous relationship		

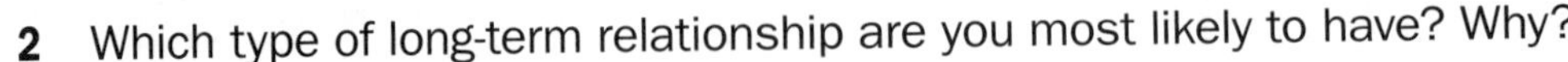

2 Which type of long-term relationship are you most likely to have? Why?

3 Do you think these types of relationships are changing? Why?

Although arranged marriages do still happen, it is now more common for young people to choose who they marry. Choosing who to marry is a very important decision. This is someone who you will probably spend the rest of your life with. You will probably live together. You might have children together and raise a family.

Each person will look for different qualities in the person they plan to marry. Many of the qualities that you might look for in a friend are the same qualities that you might look for in a marriage partner.

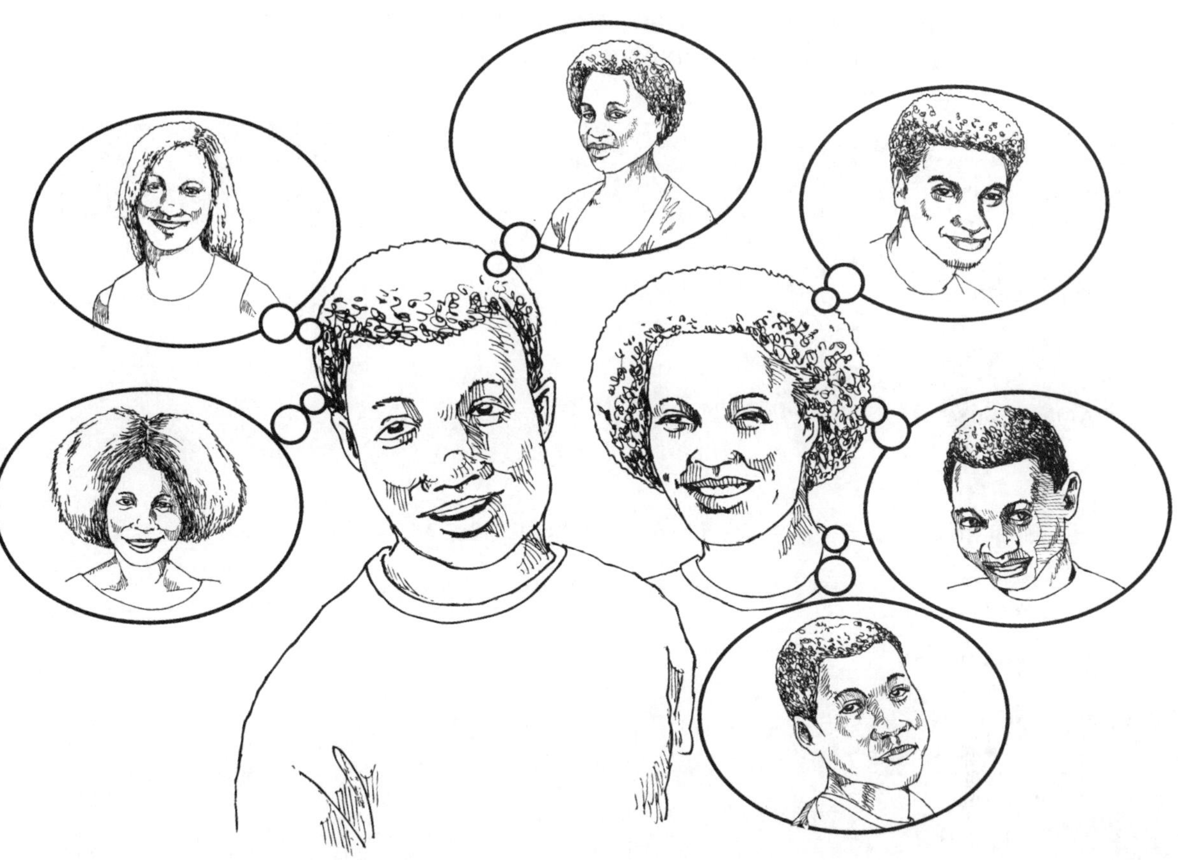

Activity 10.2 MR OR MRS RIGHT

1 Consider your answers for Activity 5.1. Are these the same qualities that you would look for in a marriage partner? Are there other qualities that you would look for in a marriage partner that you wouldn't look for in a friend?

2 Consider the following situations that married people experience. What qualities might you want in a marriage partner to share these experiences with?

Situation	Qualities that you might look for
Living together	• neatness •
Buying a house	• Do they have a job? •
Celebrating holidays	• Do they have the same beliefs as you? •
Sexual relationship	• attractive •
Having careers	• •
Caring for someone if they are sick	• •
Supporting your wantoks	• •
Having children and raising a family	• •

Even if a person has all of the qualities you might be looking for in a marriage partner, they still might not be the right person for you. It is also important that marriage partners share the same ideas about marriage and how they want to live together. It is best for couples to talk about what they want from a marriage before they get married. Couples who expect similar things from their marriage will experience less conflict.

Activity 10.3 YOUR MARRIAGE EXPECTATIONS

Knowing what you want from a marriage is an important part of choosing the person you want to marry and share your life with. The following questions will help you to think about what you expect or want from a marriage.

- Will you work? Will your partner work?
- How will you share your money?
- Do you want children? How many? When?
- How will you look after children?
- How will you share housework?
- Where will you live? In the town? In the village?
- What kind of house will you live in? An apartment? A bush material house?
- Will you spend all of your time together?
- Will you have separate interests? Separate groups of friends?
- How important is your religion to you?
- How important is faithfulness to you?
- What habits or behaviours are acceptable? Smoking? Heavy drinking?
- Will you both get an HIV test?
- How will you deal with disagreements?

Compare your marriage expectations with your friends. Do girls have different expectations than boys? Are some expectations more important than others?

Age matters

Getting married is a very important decision for two people to make. As you grow older, you develop stronger values and goals for yourself. You develop communication, negotiation and decision-making skills that reflect your values, goals and expectations. Getting married when you are too young may not give you enough time to develop these skills to make a decision that is healthy and responsible.

Some people feel ready to get married when they are in their twenties, and some people don't feel ready until they are in their thirties. Some people might never want to get married. It is important to decide what age is right for you.

Activity 10.4 YOUR ADVICE

1 With a group of mixed-sex peers, discuss these statements from young people about marriage. Are these good reasons for getting married? What advice would you give them?

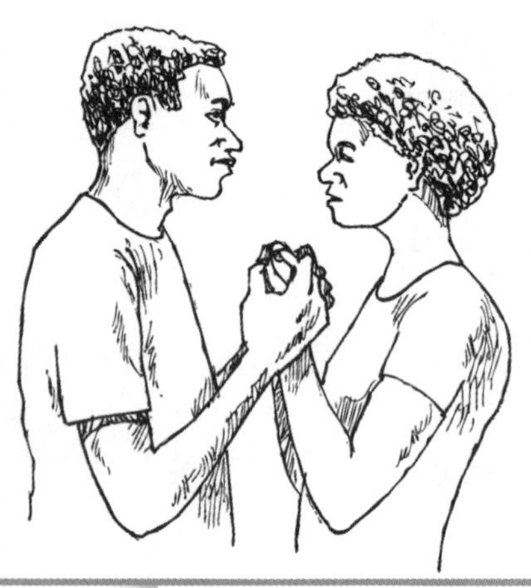

We both want to wait until we are married to have sex. We have been together for a long time and now we want to have a physical relationship.

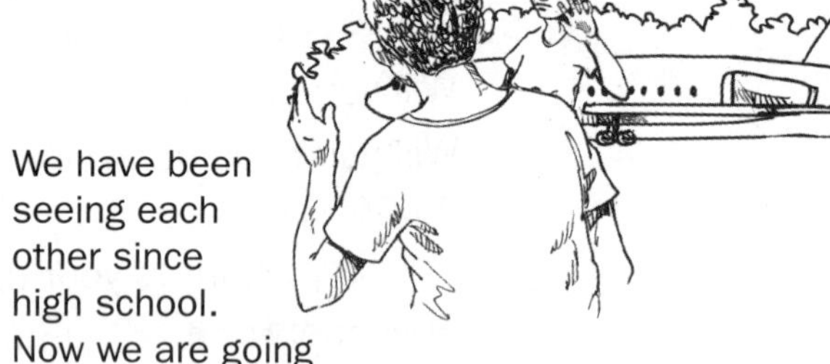

We have been seeing each other since high school. Now we are going to university in different parts of the country. Getting married will make sure we are loyal to each other.

2 Discuss the following questions in your group.

a What is an ideal age to get married? Is this different for boys and girls? Why?

b Do you have personal goals for school, a career or travel? Can you achieve these when you are married?

Decision making and conflict resolution in marriage

As with any relationship, there will be times when couples disagree about different issues. There can be many sources of stress for couples and learning how to cope with these stresses is important for having a healthy relationship.

Look at conflict resolution strategies identified in Chapters 3 and 5. These same strategies can be used by couples to resolve their differences. Some of them are listed below:

- communication
- respect
- understanding
- patience
- flexibility.

Older men and young wives

In PNG it is common for young girls to marry older men.

This can be unhealthy for a number of reasons:

- There is unequal power between the couple.
- The older man is more experienced.
- The young girl will be dependent on the man for income.
- The older man has more sexual partners.
- Often the man already has a first wife.

Activity 10.5 INTERVIEW

Identify people in your community who have been married for a long time. Interview them to learn how they have handled disagreements in their relationship.

- What were the most common things that couples disagreed about?
- How did couples resolve their disagreements?
- Did men and women have different ways to resolve their disagreements?

Discuss your findings with your peers.

Chapter 11 Parenthood

Becoming parents

Becoming a parent can be an exciting and rewarding experience. It is also a lifelong responsibility that requires commitment and cooperation.

Parents must be prepared to provide for the many needs that children have. Some of these needs can be provided for with love, care and attention. Other needs require money and security.

Activity 11.1 ROLES AND RESPONSIBILITIES OF PARENTS

What are the roles and responsibilities of parents? Discuss this question with your peers.

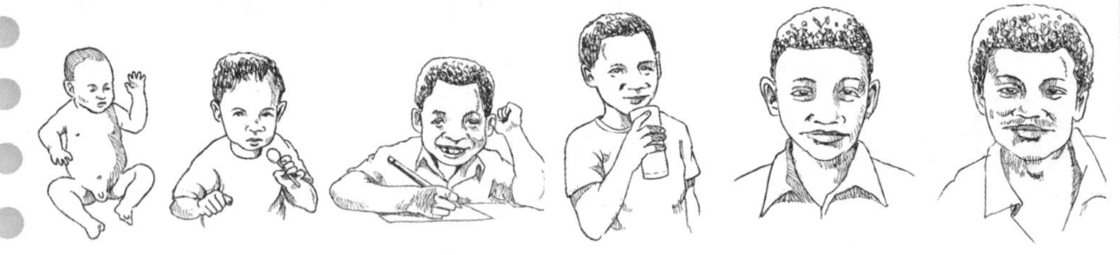

Roles of parents	Responsibilities of parents
• understanding • caring	• to ensure access to health facilities, vaccinations • to provide food, clothing and shelter
•	•
•	•
•	•

Becoming a parent will change your life in many different ways. It is important for you to decide if having children and raising a family is something that you want to do.

Activity 11.2 BRAINSTORM

There are many reasons people choose to become a parent or not to become a parent. In a mixed-sex group, brainstorm different reasons.

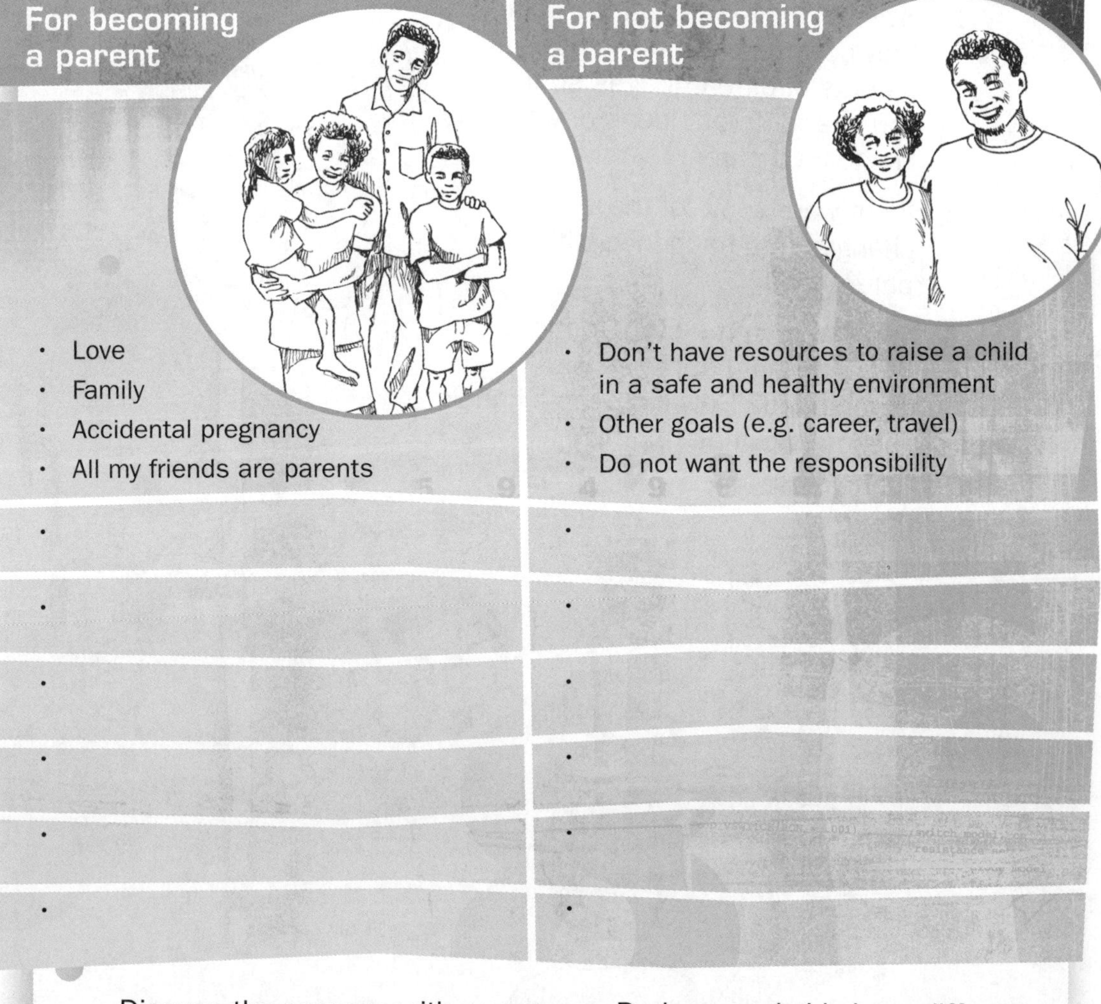

For becoming a parent	For not becoming a parent
• Love • Family • Accidental pregnancy • All my friends are parents	• Don't have resources to raise a child in a safe and healthy environment • Other goals (e.g. career, travel) • Do not want the responsibility
•	•
•	•
•	•
•	•
•	•
•	•

Discuss the reasons with your group. Do boys and girls have different reasons for becoming or not becoming a parent?
Are some of these reasons stronger than other ones?

Preparing for parenthood

Choosing to have children and to raise a family is a very big decision for couples to make. Children have many needs that require time, attention and resources. It is the parents' responsibility to provide for these needs.

Activity 11.3 INTERVIEW

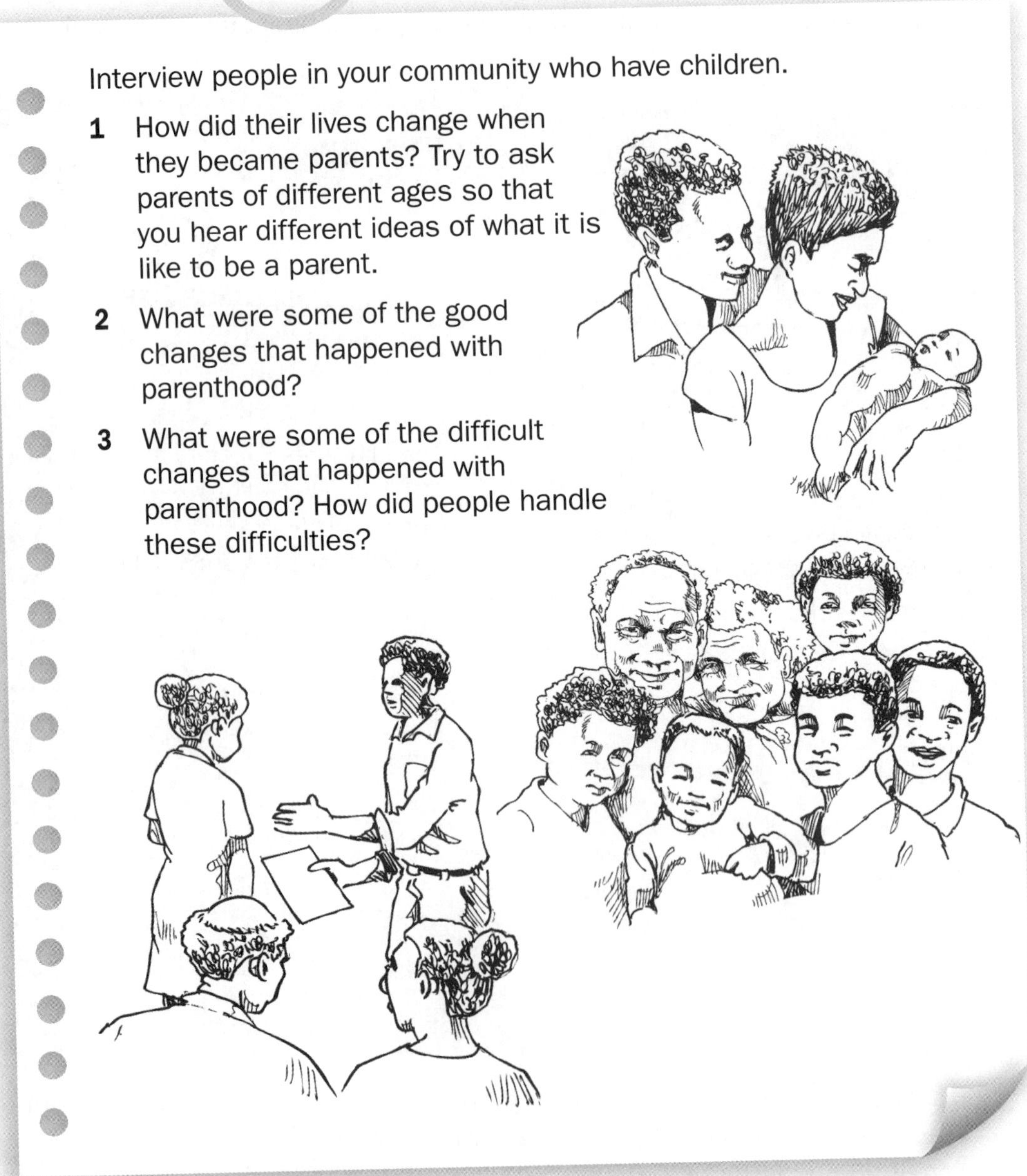

Interview people in your community who have children.

1. How did their lives change when they became parents? Try to ask parents of different ages so that you hear different ideas of what it is like to be a parent.
2. What were some of the good changes that happened with parenthood?
3. What were some of the difficult changes that happened with parenthood? How did people handle these difficulties?

Before becoming parents, couples should talk about their goals and expectations for parenthood. This will help them to decide if they are ready to become parents, and when the right time might be for them to have children. Talking openly and honestly about your thoughts and feelings about parenthood will help you to become stronger and better parents. Here are some questions that couples can think about.

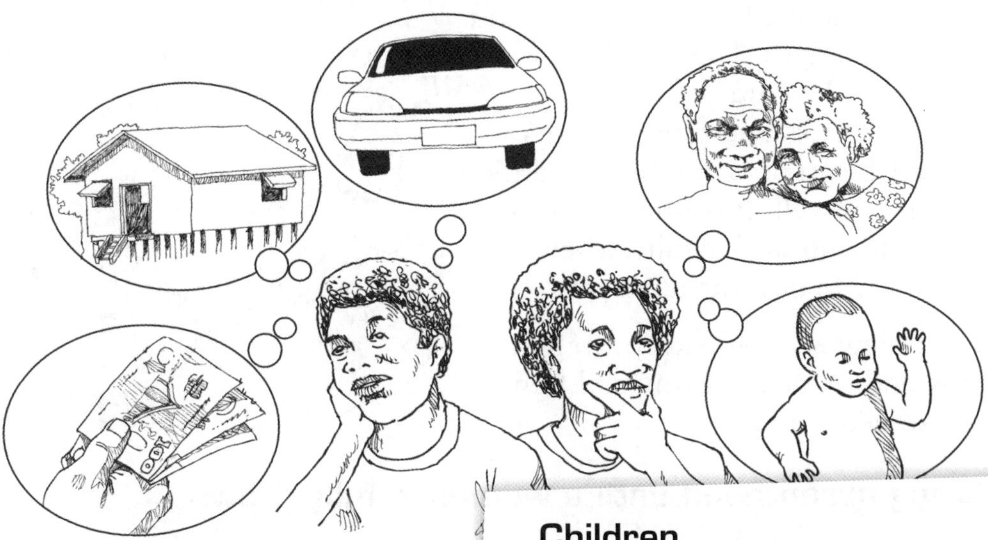

Children

- Do we both want children?
- How many children do we want?
- Do we want to have our own children?
- Do we want to adopt a child?

Relationship

- Do we have a strong relationship?
- Do we love and respect each other?
- Do we communicate well?
- How do we handle disagreements?

Health and behaviour

- Do we have healthy behaviours and lifestyles?
- Are we healthy?
- Are we old enough to have children?
- Are we too old to have children?

Supporting children

- Do we have a steady source of income?
- Do we have a garden to provide some of our food?
- Will we have money for school fees?
- Do we have a safe home?
- Do we already have other children? Will we be able to support another child?

Other support

- Do we have the support of our families?
- Do we live close to our families?
- Do we have the support of our church?
- Do we have other people who can support us?

Impacts of pregnancy on women

Pregnancy can be a very happy time for a woman and her partner. They will be excited about the arrival of a baby. However, during pregnancy, women experience many different physical and emotional changes. Their bodies grow and stretch. They may experience morning sickness and mood swings. Giving birth can be a painful and difficult experience as well. It is important to consider the mother's health when you are planning to become a parent.

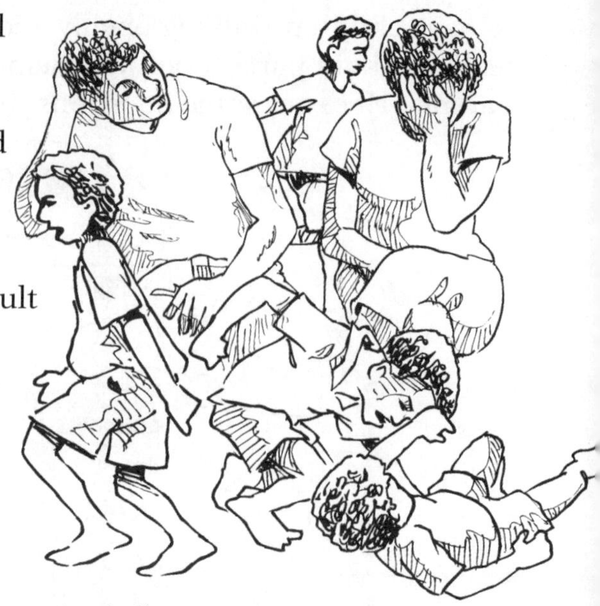

Some strategies to help keep women healthy and to have healthy children are presented below.

Delaying parenthood until a woman is fully grown

Pregnancy and childbirth are very demanding on a woman physically and emotionally.

Although a woman is physically able to have children when she is 12 or 13 years old, at this age her body is still growing and developing. Becoming a parent when a woman is too young can be harmful for the mother and the child.

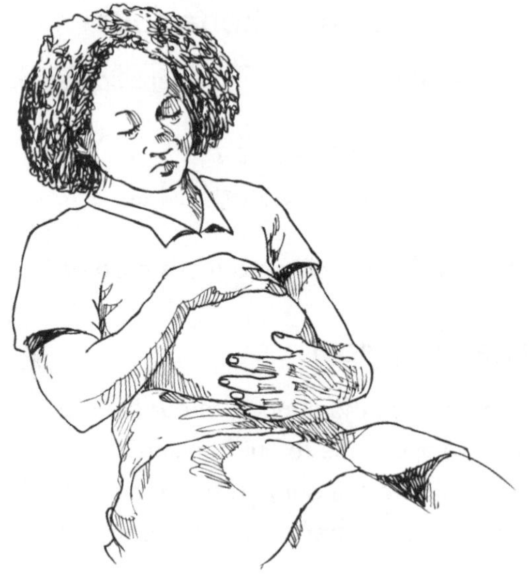

A young woman may:

- experience more difficult pregnancy and childbirth
- have to stop her education, giving up opportunities for further study, career and a way to support her family in the future
- have a family that does not support her and the early pregnancy, causing conflict and stress
- have a relationship that isn't strong enough or ready to handle such a responsibility.

Planning the number of children

In your grandparent's generation, couples used to have many children and families were very large. In more recent times, couples have been having fewer children. Pregnancy and childbirth are very demanding on a woman. In PNG, most women do not have access to health care services that offer services for complicated pregnancies and child delivery.

Also, the more children a couple have, the more children they have to care for and support. Parents should consider their ability to provide for all the needs of their children when they decide how many children they would like to have.

Spacing children

Women who have too many children too close together risk their health. Pregnancy, childbirth, breastfeeding and caring for infants cause physical strains on women's bodies. Women must have enough time between pregnancies to allow for their bodies to recover and return to health.

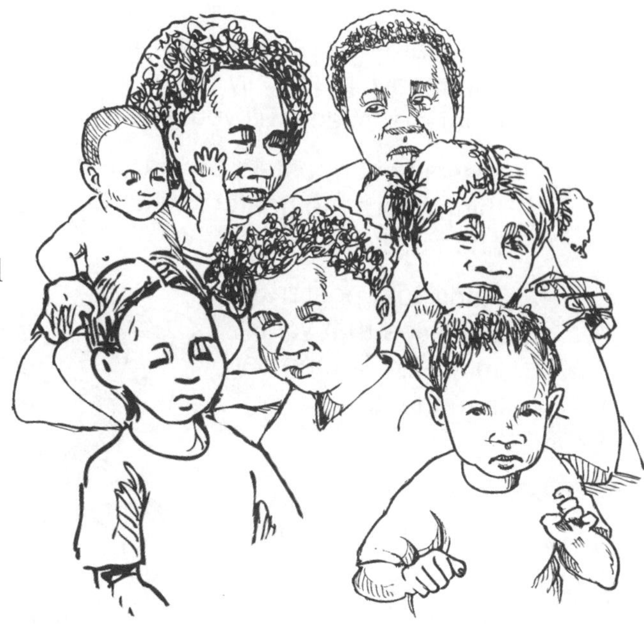

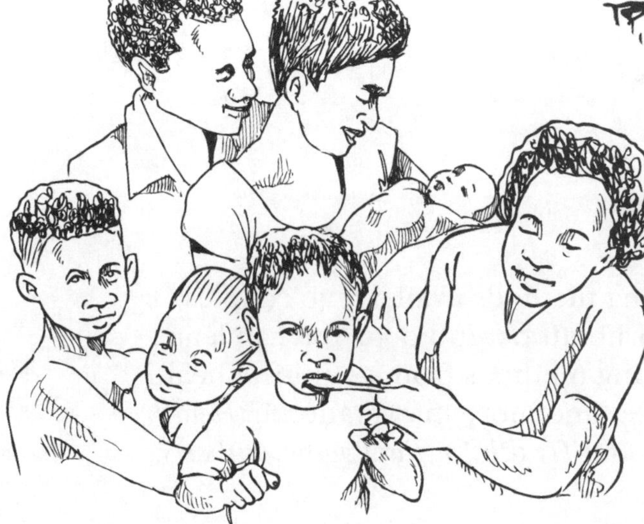

Delaying parenthood until a woman is fully grown, having small families and allowing enough time between children are all strategies that will help to keep women healthy. They will also improve the health of children and families.

Adoption

Adoption is another way to become a parent. Couples who cannot have children or want to expand their family without putting the woman at risk often choose to adopt. In PNG, it is very common for children to live away from their parents, with other family members.

Activity 11.4 CAMPAIGN

Make an awareness poster for young people who are thinking about having a family. What messages will you give to young men? What messages will you give to young women?

Present your posters to your friends and peers. What do they think about the poster? What do they think about safe parenthood and family planning?

Hang your posters in places that young men and women can see them.

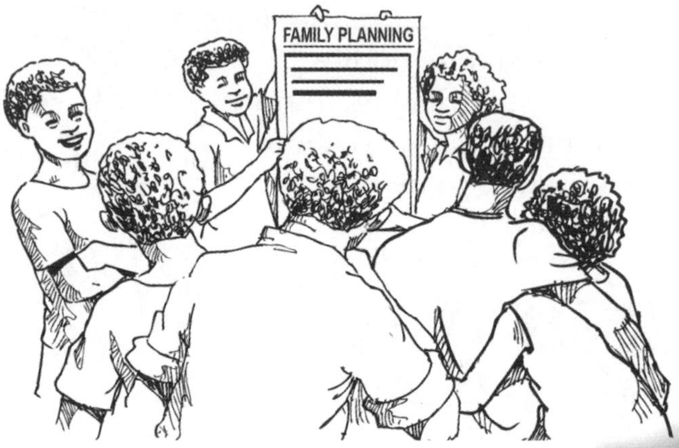

There are a range of family planning methods available to couples to help them make healthy choices about parenthood. You can learn more about different family planning methods from your local health care worker or teacher. You can also find more information in *Health for the Pacific: HIV/AIDS and STIs* and *Health for the Pacific: Puberty, Reproduction and Sexuality*.

Chapter 12 Changing relationships

Throughout your life you will have many different relationships. Some relationships will last for a very long time, and some will only last for a short time. Some relationships will be very strong, and some will be casual. Learning how to handle changing relationships in a mature and respectful manner will help you to have a happy life.

Why relationships change

Relationships can change for many different reasons. These include:

- growing older
- moving
- becoming a parent
- falling in love, falling out of love
- changing interests
- changing feelings
- different goals and expectations
- illness and disability
- death.

When relationships change, people often experience strong feelings and emotions. These can be happy feelings, such as in the start of a new friendship or becoming a parent. These can also be sad or painful feelings, such as when a relationship breaks up or someone passes away. All of these emotions are natural. It is important to learn how to handle these emotions.

Activity 12.1 CHANGING RELATIONSHIPS

Think of a time when you experienced a change in your relationship.

- What caused the change?
- How did you feel?
- What did you do to help you understand the change?

How and when relationships change varies from relationship to relationship. It is important to remember that you have the right to make decisions about your relationships. You can decide which relationships you want to maintain and which you want to end.

If you are in a relationship that is unhealthy, you can take steps to change or end the relationship. This can be difficult to do, but if you find yourself in this situation, it is important to think about your goals and values. Ending an unhealthy relationship may be difficult and painful for a little while, but it will help you to have a healthier and happier life in the long run. Having a strong network of friends and family to support you can help to make this experience easier.

Changing family relationships

As children grow and develop, their relationship with their family changes. The way a person's relationship with their family can change depends on their age, sex, culture and religion. There might be changes in a person's roles and responsibilities, their independence, their freedom and their contribution to family decisions.

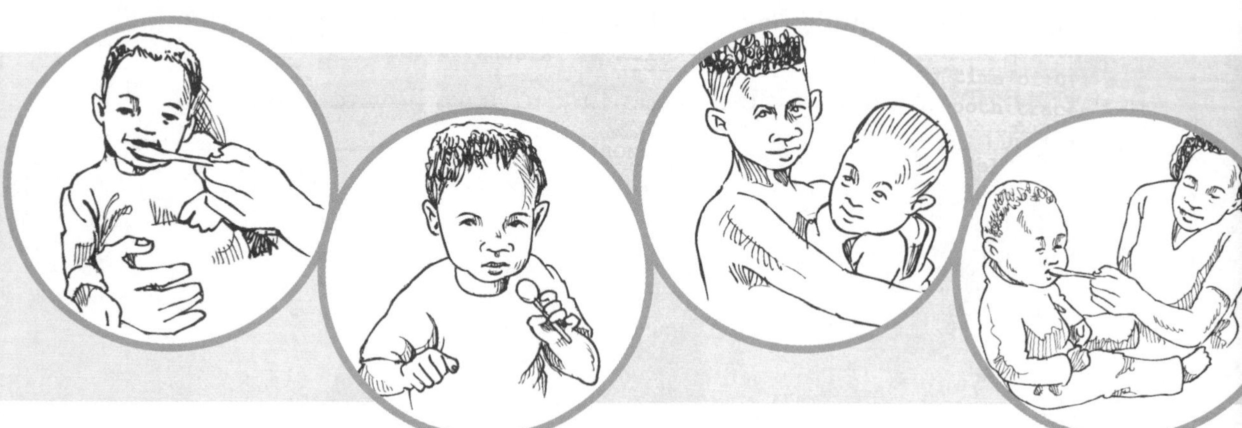

Activity 12.2 MY CHANGING FAMILY RELATIONSHIP

Complete the following table for different stages in a person's life. How does a person's relationship change in their family at each stage? Is this different for boys and girls? Compare your answers with your friends' answers.

Age	Responsibilities	Independence	Decision making	Contribution to house and family well-being
0–5 years				
6–10 years				
11–14 years				
15–18 years				
19–24 years				
24+ years				

Changing friendships

Throughout your life, you will meet many people and you will develop many friendships. You may not always be friends with the same people that you are friends with now. The people you are friends with now may not be the same people you were friends with when you were younger.

As you grow older, your values, interests and character change. These changes happen for many different reasons and can be influenced by many different factors, including age, sex, education, and cultural and religious beliefs.

Death

Sadly, relationships end when someone dies. This may cause many strong emotions, such as sadness, anger and loss. In PNG cultures there are traditions that help people say goodbye to those who have passed away. Being a part of these celebrations and traditions is a good way to deal with the loss of a close friend or family member.

Activity 12.3 JOURNAL ENTRY

Have you ever lost someone close to you? How did you feel?

Was there a ceremony or funeral for the person who died? Was it a traditional ceremony?

Write a journal entry about a time when someone close to you passed away. Describe how you felt. Describe the funeral ceremonies.

If you have never lost someone, interview a friend or family member about their experience.

Activity 12.4 INTERVIEW

Different cultures have different ways of remembering and honouring people who pass away. Many of these traditions are still practised today. Some of them have changed and some of them have been forgotten. How people celebrate those who pass away is a very important part of your culture and history.

Interview people in your community about how they celebrate and remember people who have passed away.

- What traditions do they have?
- Is there singing? Dancing? Eating?
- What do people in your community believe about what happens to a person after they die?
- Have these traditions and practices changed?

Ending a relationship

Ending a friendship or romantic relationship is upsetting and difficult. This is a person you have liked and shared many experiences with. But perhaps you are not getting on well now or you are moving on to a different part of your life. Maybe the relationship is becoming unhealthy.

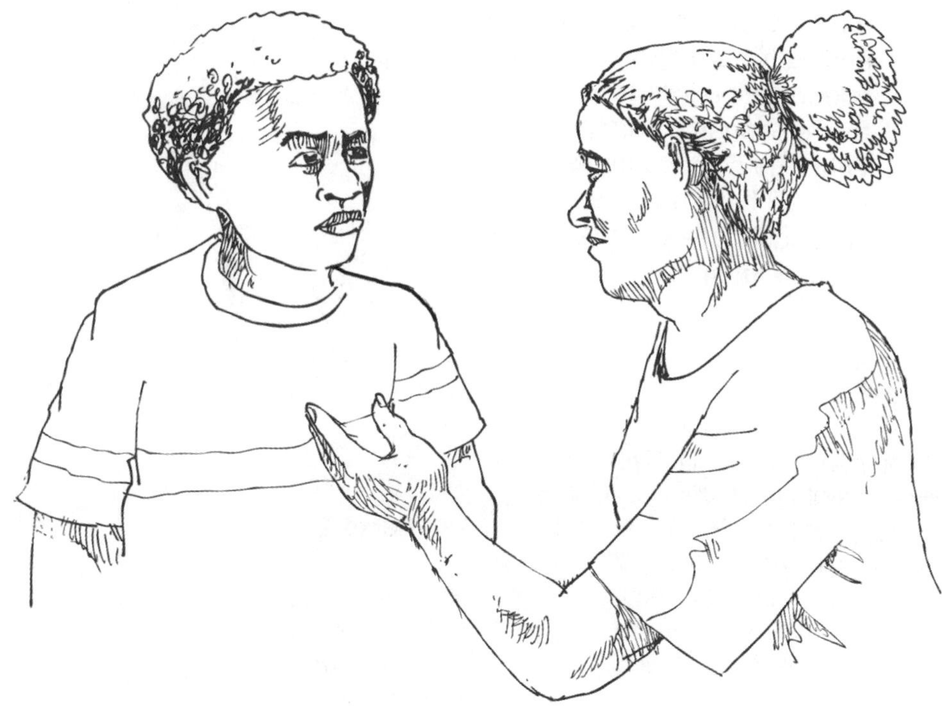

Here are some tips for ending a relationship in a sensible and healthy way.

- Think about what you will say and why you want to finish the relationship.
- Plan for the consequences – what will you do next?
- Once you have made a decision, tell the person quickly.
- Tell the person in person, face-to-face.
- If you think they might become angry, make sure you choose a safe place.
- Be honest and explain your decision.
- Stick to your decision.

Activity 12.5 HAPPY ENDINGS

1 For each scenario, write a happy ending (where the person ending the relationship follows the tips on the previous page) and a sad ending (where they don't use their relationship skills to end the relationship safely). Write the conversations they will have and the consequences of these conversations.

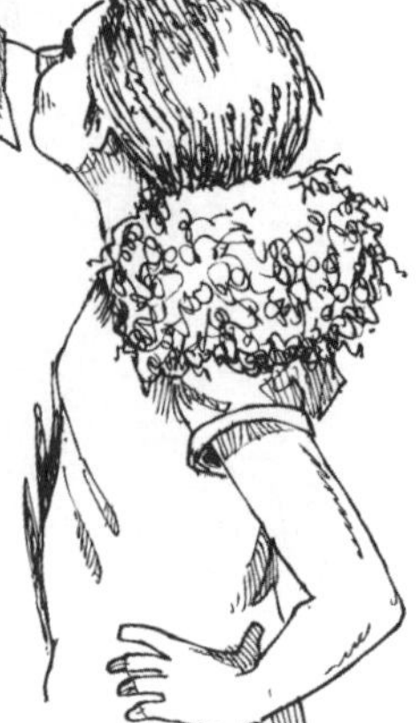

Scenario 1

Marshall and Judy have been boyfriend and girlfriend since the start of high school. Judy feels that Marshall is not very sensible and spends too much time with his friends getting into trouble. They keep arguing. She decides to tell him that their relationship is over.

Scenario 2

Naomi and Joseph have been seeing each other since primary school. He has moved away from the village and has fallen in love with one of his workmates. He needs to tell Naomi that he wants to end their relationship so he can start a new one.

Scenario 3

Thadius and Rachel have been married for four years and have two children. Thadius has started drinking and lost his job. He gets angry a lot and has started beating Rachel. Quickly, she decides to leave him. She is scared for herself and her children.

2 Now write a scenario of your own.

Chapter 13 My goals

It is important to have a good understanding of what you want and what you expect from your relationships. Knowing this will help you to understand what you are comfortable with and what acceptable and unacceptable behaviour is. It will help you to make healthy decisions about your relationships.

Activity 13.1 MY PERSONAL GOALS

Consider what you have read and learned throughout this book. What are your goals for your own relationships? What will you do to keep healthy and safe in your relationships?

Complete these statements with your own goals.

Values I look for in other people are ...

I am a good friend/partner/sibling/child because ....

The most important relationships to me now are ...

Relationships that I would like to have in the future are ...

In my relationships, I expect people to ...

My role model for healthy relationships is ... because ...

In my relationships acceptable behaviours are ...

In my relationships unacceptable behaviours are ...

My rights in relationships are ...

My responsibilities in relationships are ...

In my community and life these things put me at risk of
unhealthy relationships ...
and this is what I will do about it ...

If I have a girlfriend or boyfriend I will keep myself and them safe by ...
I will not have sex until ...
I will go to ... for advice and support because ...
I will not get married until ... because ...
My future family will be this size ... because ...
This is how I want to be treated by any boyfriend or girlfriend ... and this is how I will treat them ...
I will use these strategies to resolve conflict ... I will never do this ... to resolve conflict.

If you need more information about relationships

Relationships are an important part of everybody's life. Having happy, healthy relationships based on respect and trust will allow you to lead a happy and productive life. Learning more about healthy relationships and knowing who you can speak to for good advice will help you to develop skills and attitudes to develop your own healthy relationships.

Sources of information could include:

- parents and family
- community leaders
- teachers
- trained school-based counsellors and guidance officers
- trained peer educators
- textbooks and health leaflets
- special telephone helplines or websites for young people
- health workers
- NGOs which work with young people like Save the Children
- peers
- elders and churches.

Other sources of information are shown on the following page.

Good books about personal development

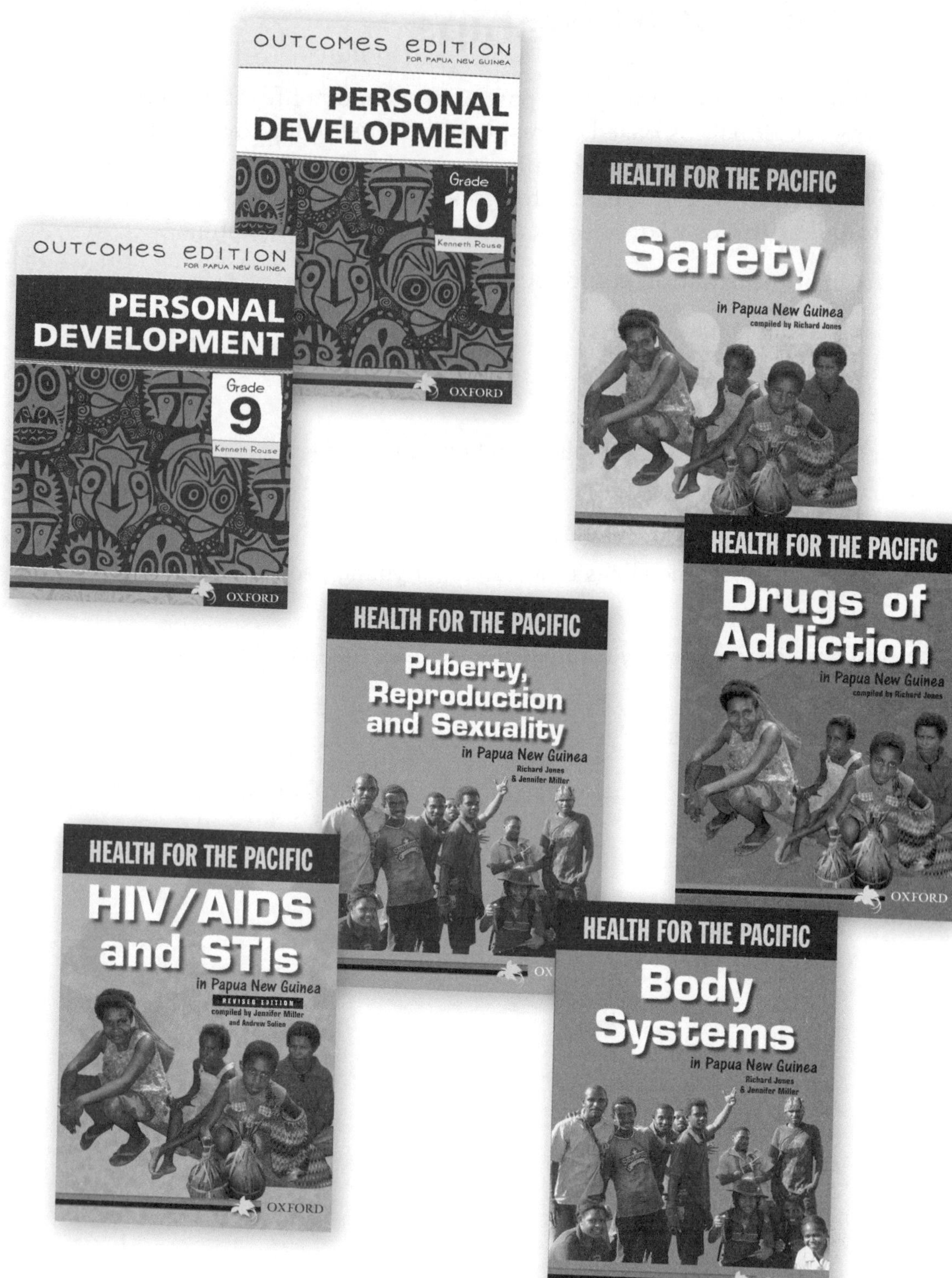

Good websites about young people's relationships

Child and teen health information **www.cyh.com**

Family planning information **www.brook.org.uk**

Puberty, peer pressure and sexual health for young people **www.likeitis.org.au**

Accurate health information about sexual practices for young people **www.scarleteen.com**

Papua New Guinea helplines

Marie Stopes sexual health helpline for young people
8am–10pm, seven days a week, free
7200 5314

BAHA helpline for HIV and AIDS
Seven days a week, free
7200 2242

Organisations who work with young people in PNG

- Save the Children in PNG
- Marie Stopes
- Scouts
- Girl Guides
- UNICEF
- Anglicare StopAIDS
- Childfund
- Pathfinder
- Susu Mama
- many churches
- Church organisations such as Caritas and ADRA
- Guidance Branch, Department of Education, and all school-based counsellors.

You can find their contact details in the phone book or on the Internet.

Glossary

acceptable behaviour
behaviour which does not cause someone any harm

adolescence
the time during puberty when children become adults; the social and physical changes during puberty

conflict resolution
solving a disagreement in a peaceful way

peer educator
a person who provides accurate information and support to someone of their own age, sex or interests

peers
people who are the same age or sex as you or share similar interests

puberty
the period of time when a child matures and develops into an adult (physically, sexually, mentally)

rape
forced sex

relationship
the social link between two people

role model
a person whose behaviour sets a good example to others

self esteem
how a person feels about themselves

sexual abuse
forced sexual behaviour

sugar daddy
an older man who uses power, money and influence to attract younger women

unacceptable behaviour
behaviour that causes harm or offence